The Menstrual Cycle and Physical Activity

Edited by
Jacqueline L. Puhl, PhD
United States Olympic Committee
Sports Medicine Division
and
C. Harmon Brown, MD
California State University, Hayward

Proceedings of the
seminar held February 24-26, 1984
at the Olympic Training Center,
Colorado Springs, Colorado under
sponsorship of the U.S. Olympic Committee
Sports Medicine Council in cooperation
with Tampax Incorporated

Human Kinetics Publishers, Inc.
Champaign, Illinois

Library of Congress Cataloging-in-Publication Data
Main entry under title:

The Menstrual cycle and physical activity.

Proceedings of the Symposium on the Menstrual Cycle
and Physical Activity, held Feb. 1984 in Colorado
Springs, Colo.
Includes bibliographies and index.
1. Women athletes—Physiology—Congresses.
2. Menstruation disorders—Congresses. 3. Exercise—
Physiological aspects—Congresses. 4. Menstrual cycle—
Congresses. I. Puhl, Jacqueline L., 1940-
II. Brown, C. Harmon, 1930-   . III. Symposium on
the Menstrual Cycle and Physical Activity (1984 :
Colorado Springs, Colo.) [DNLM: 1. Menstrual Cycle—
congresses. 2. Menstruation Disorders—congresses.
3. Physical Education and Training—congresses.
WP 550 M548 1984]
RC1218.W65M46   1986   618.1'75'0088796   85-22427
ISBN 0-87322-026-9

Developmental Editor: Susan Wilmoth, PhD
Production Director: Sara Chilton
Copyeditor: Carol Poto
Text Design: Julie Szamocki
Typesetter: Sandra Meier
Text Layout: Cyndy Barnes
Cover Design and Layout: Chu Usadel
Printed by: Braun-Brumfield

ISBN 0-87322-026-9

Printed in the United States of America

10 9 8 7 6 5 4 3 2 1

Human Kinetics Publishers, Inc.
Box 5076, Champaign, IL 61820

Contents

Acknowledgments

We are indebted to Tampax Incorporated and especially to Dr. Clayton Thomas, director of Medical Affairs for Tampax, for their generous and enthusiastic support of this symposium. We are also indebted to the many experts who contributed their research and knowledge to the symposium, and to the staff of the USOC Sports Medicine Division of Education Services who contributed greatly in such efforts as planning and logistics to make the symposium a success and to ensure that publication of the proceedings became a reality.

We encourage financial support for future research so that we can answer athletes, parents, and coaches with greater assurance when they present questions about the short-term and long-term potential effects of exercise.

Jacqueline L. Puhl, PhD

C. Harmon Brown, MD

Preface

The explosive growth of women in sport over the past 15 years has raised numerous questions concerning the physiological adaptations and health of women participating in sport. One of the most important areas of interest and concern is the effect of training on menstrual cycle function. There is increasing evidence that menstrual cycle alterations occur with some types of training. Research on physical activity and the menstrual cycle has progressed through descriptive, epidemiological research toward attempts to understand potential causes and their interactions and hormonal mechanisms involved in menstrual dysfunction.

In recent years, some research has focused on hormonal alterations associated with acute and chronic exercise. A number of current investigators are providing information on effects of long-term strenuous training on bone density. Implications of such findings and future directions for osteoporosis and bone fracture studies need to be clarified. Ultimately, research on the physiological effects of exercise and training on women must deal with the reversibility of any menstrual dysfunction that may occur in certain individuals and with the prevention of any negative effects associated with long-term strenuous training.

The United States Olympic Committee is conscious of its responsibility to help provide for the health and well-being of all amateur athletes in the United States and to contribute to the body of knowledge concerning the health of exercising Americans. Through seminars, workshops, and symposia, the Sports Medicine Council and Division bring together outstanding scholars to share and disseminate information about various medical aspects of sport as well as to germinate new ideas for future research. The purpose of this February

Symposium on the Menstrual Cycle and Physical Activity was to provide state-of-the-art information about

1. prevalence of menstrual cycle alterations associated with training;
2. identification of associated factors and theories of menstrual dysfunction;
3. hormonal alterations associated with exercise and training of women in sport
4. the relationship between strenuous training and bone density in young women; and
5. methodological and technological problems involved with research on the menstrual cycle.

Additional questions of concern to athletes and parents include long-term effects of altered menstrual cycles on reproductive capability and health and the integrity of the skeletal system.

The symposium format involved the presentation of a major topic followed by comments from a predesigned reactor. The reactions provided supporting as well as contrasting points of view and acted as a catalyst for the ensuing discussion. In a prevailing atmosphere of sharing and exchanging, the format of presentation, reaction, and discussion helped identify areas of concern and provide motivation for future research.

Jacqueline L. Puhl, PhD

C. Harmon Brown, MD

1

Historical Perspectives of Research on Physical Activity and the Menstrual Cycle

Elizabeth Renwick Baker
The Milton S. Hershey Medical Center

Over the past 15 years, more women have begun to participate in strenuous endurance sports. In addition, the level of competition and vigorous training requirements far exceed those seen in the past, although it is difficult to determine women's participation in athletic events in early history. Only the Spartan society, because of its belief that well-conditioned women made better childbearers, encouraged women to pursue vigorous physical activity. In the United States, sporting events for women were established by German teachers who had emigrated following the German Revolution of 1849. First came gymnastics (1859), followed later by tennis (1875) and crew (1880). In 1894 the sport of basketball was instituted at Smith College and remained a women's event until 1910. In the 1912 Olympics, women entered many events. Unfortunately, in the 1920s, sports for women were viewed as unladylike and physically and emotionally harmful, thereby ending female participation in a wide variety of sports. This trend was not reversed until the 1950s when the attitude that vigorous physical activity is unfeminine was challenged. People now realize that women are physically and emotionally capable of participating in strenuous sports activity (Hunter, 1980). Today over 6 million women run, 1 million play soccer, and over 1/3 of high school athletes are female (Speroff, 1982). This continuous increase in the number of women athletes has prompted investigators to study the effects of vigorous physical activity on the menstrual cycle and on reproduction.

Sports and the Menstrual Cycle

Evidence suggests a causal relationship between increased strenuous athletic activity and a higher incidence of delayed menarche and menstrual dysfunction. Erdelyi (1962), Malina (1978), and Prokop (cited in Erdelyi, 1976) have noted a higher incidence of either delayed menarche or subsequent menstrual dysfunction in girls undergoing intense athletic activity prior to menarche. According to Malina, menarche was attained latest in Olympic athletes and earliest in nonathletes. Frisch et al. (1981) found that in premenarche-trained swimmers and runners, menarche was delayed 5 months for each year of training before menarche. In contrast, Erdelyi (1962) found no change in menarche but noted a higher incidence of later menstrual dysfunction in those girls with intensive premenarcheal athletic training compared with the general Hungarian population. Feicht, Johnson, Martin, Sparkes, and Wagner (1978) have not found either of these cases to be true. Delayed menarche and subsequent menstrual dysfunction are also found in ballet dancers who undergo intense prepubertal training and are highly motivated to maintain low body weights (Frisch, Wyshak, & Vincent, 1980; Warren, 1980).

The American College of Sports Medicine has reported that approximately 1/3 of competitive female long-distance runners between ages 12 and 45 experience periods of amenorrhea or oligomenorrhea (Dale, Gerlach, Martin, & Alexander, 1979; Dale, Gerlach, & Wilhite, 1979). The reported incidence of menstrual dysfunction in athletes has ranged from 0% to 50% (Dale et al., 1979; Kabisch, cited in Erdelyi, 1976). Rougier and Linquette (1962) found varied effects of exercise on the menstrual cycles of physical education students; likewise, Kabisch, in evaluating East German athletes, found few incidences of amenorrhea. In contrast, Erdelyi (1976), who studied top caliber female athletes, and Zhanel (1971), who studied female fencers, found a 10% to 12% incidence of menstrual dysfunction. In a study comparing collegiate swimmers, cyclists, and runners, the incidence of amenorrhea for swimmers and cyclists was approximately 12%, whereas that for runners was 25.7% (Feicht et al., 1978). However, among recreational runners in one survey, only 7.9% reported amenorrhea since the onset of training (Speroff & Redwine, 1980). From these studies the incidence of menstrual dysfunction appears to vary directly with the degree of physical effort exerted during training and competition.

Risk Factors

From past research, a variety of risk factors which may predispose the athlete to amenorrhea have been identified. These include irregular menses prior to sports participation, young age or nulliparity, stress, and weight loss or alteration in percent body fat. Schwartz et al. (1981) found that amenorrheic runners had a higher incidence of irregular menses prior to running than runners who did not develop amenorrhea; however, Erdelyi (1976), Speroff and Redwine (1980), and Baker (1981) found no increased incidence of prior menstrual irregularity in those athletes who became amenorrheic as compared to those who maintained regular menstrual cycles.

Several studies suggest that younger athletes, under age 25, may be more prone to develop amenorrhea as a consequence of their sport participation (Baker, 1981; Speroff & Redwine, 1980). Nulliparity may also influence the runner's susceptibility to menstrual dysfunction. Dale et al. (1979) noted that only 21% of the multiparous runners studied developed amenorrhea, whereas 51% of the nulliparous group became amenorrheic. This simple association between prior pregnancy and protection against amenorrhea may not reflect cause and effect because other factors may be involved.

The role of stress and energy expenditure is difficult to evaluate; however, the observation that athletes have a higher incidence of amenorrhea while participating in strenuous sports raises the possibility of a stress-related phenomenon (Harris, 1978; Wentz, 1980). Amenorrheic runners were similar to menstrually regular runners in levels of depression, hypochondriasis, anxiety, and obsessive/compulsive tendencies; however, they did associate more stress with their running program (Schwartz et al., 1981). Chronic physical or emotional stress may produce a state of either hypoestrogenic amenorrhea or euestrogenic anovulation (Shangold, 1980).

The effects on the menstrual cycle of mileage run per week are controversial. Several studies (Feicht et al., 1978; Foreman, cited in Dale et al., 1979; Shangold, Freeman, Thysen, & Gatz, 1979) have noted a significant correlation between miles run per week and amenorrhea or luteal phase defect; other studies (Baker, Mathur, Kirk, & Williamson, 1981; Speroff & Redwine, 1980) have not found this to be an important factor in the development of secondary amenorrhea.

Secondary amenorrhea can also result from excessive weight loss, alteration of percent body fat, and perhaps from altered dietary intake. The data from past studies suggest that a particular body composition may play an important role in the regulation of the menstrual cycle (Frisch & McArthur, 1974). Several studies (Dale et al., 1979; Frisch & McArthur, 1974; Schwartz et al., 1981; Speroff & Redwine, 1980; Wentz, 1980) have noted that amenorrheic runners are more likely to have lower initial body weight for height, greater weight loss since the onset of training, and a lower percent body fat than menstrually regular runners. However, two other studies (Baker et al., 1981; Feicht et al., 1978) found comparable mean height, weight, and weight loss for amenorrheic and menstrually regular runners. With regard to diet, amenorrheic runners consumed more calories per day than did other runners or controls (Schwartz, 1981), but fewer of these calories were derived from proteins. Perhaps alterations in body composition or diet combined with stress may predispose some athletes to the development of amenorrhea.

Hormonal Investigations

Numerous studies have evaluated the effects of exercise and athletic training on levels of steroid hormones, prolactin, gonadotropins, neurotransmitters, and prostaglandins and have obtained a variety of results depending on the type of exercise and the timing of the samples (Baker et al., 1981; Baker et al., 1983; Bonen et al., 1979; Boyden et al., 1982; Boyden et al., 1983; Brisson, Volle, DeCarufel, Desharnis, & Tanaka, 1980; Dale et al., 1979; Demers, Harrison, Halbert, & Santen, cited in Grunby, 1981; Jurkowski, Jones, Walker, Younglai, & Sutton, 1978; Shangold et al., 1979; Shangold et al., 1981). In general, estradiol, prolactin, luteinizing hormone, and the adrenal androgens increased immediately after exercise, as did dopamine, epinephrine, norepinephrine, and the prostaglandins. However, in studies done 12 to 24 hours after exercise, estradiol, prolactin, luteinizing hormone, and progesterone were decreased in amenorrheic runners.

Reversibility and Osteoporosis

Preliminary studies have shown decreased bone mineral content in some amenorrheic hyperprolactinemic women (Schlechte, Sherman, & Martin, 1983) and also in some nonmenstruating female athletes (Gonzalez, 1982). On the basis of this initial data, amenorrheic athletes may be at risk for premature osteoporosis and may benefit from supplemental estrogen. Our own data at Hershey suggest an increased risk of injury for amenorrheic runners, which may be avoided by the use of oral contraceptives. However, more studies need to be done to verify this association.

Many amenorrheic female athletes are concerned about their future reproductive ability and whether or not exercise-related amenorrhea will be reversible. Several studies in the literature are reassuring:

1. Amenorrheic rowers resumed menses after the close of the rowing season (Erdelyi, 1962).
2. When training was interrupted, amenorrheic ballet dancers and amenorrheic runners often resumed menses within several months (Foreman, 1967; Warren, 1980).
3. Young girl swimmers had normal reproductive functions 10 years after discontinuing strenuous training (Eriksson et al., 1978).
4. In a study by Stager et al. (1984), ex-athletes who had indicated altered menses during training reported resumption of normal cyclic menses

within a mean of 1.7 months after training was halted, and amenorrhea appeared not to persist longer than 6 months after cessation of training.

Conclusion

How many amenorrheic athletes have a reversible problem and will be able to achieve pregnancy when they decrease their level of training? Each athlete probably has an individual set point for the development of amenorrhea, and this threshold may be modified by a variety of factors. Many factors have been implicated in the onset of exercise-related amenorrhea and estimates of the incidence of this phenomenon vary widely. Studies have been done to attempt to define the short- and long-term consequences of strenuous exercise (Baker, 1981) and at present we assume that these alterations in the menstrual cycle are reversible. However, long-term investigations are still needed to further define the mechanisms, risk factors, and consequences of athletic amenorrhea.

References

Åstrand, P., Eriksson, B., Nylander, I., Engstrom, L., Karlberg, P., Saltin, B., & Thoren, C. (1963). Girl swimmers. *Acta Paediatrica Scandinavica*, (Suppl. 147), 33.

Baker, E.R., Mathur, R.S., Kirk, R.F., & Williamson, H.O. (1981). Female runners and secondary amenorrhea: Correlation with age, parity, mileage and plasma hormonal and sex-hormone-binding globulin concentrations. *Fertility and Sterility*, **36**, 183.

Baker, E.R. (1981). Menstrual dysfunction and hormonal status in athletic women: A review. *Fertility and Sterility*, **36**, 691.

Baker, E.R., Mathur, R.S., Kirk, R.F., Landgrebe, S., Moody, L., & Williamson, H.O. (1982). Plasma gonadotropins, prolactin, and steroid hormone concentrations in female runners immediately after a long distance run. *Fertility and Sterility*, **38**, 38.

Bonen, A., Ling, W.Y., MacIntyre, K.P., Neil, R., McGrail, J.C., & Belcastro, A.N. (1979). Effects of exercise on the serum concentrations of FSH, LH, progesterone, and estradiol. *European Journal of Applied Physiology*, **42**, 15.

Bonen, A., Belcastro, A.N., Ling, W.Y., & Simpson, A.A. (1981). Profiles of selected hormones during menstrual cycles of teenage athletes. *Journal of Applied Physiology*, **50**, 545.

Boyden, T.W., Pamenter, R.W., Grosso, D., Stanforth, P., Rotkis, T., & Wilmore, J.H. (1982). Prolactin responses, menstrual cycles, and body composition of women runners. *Journal of Clinical Endocrinology and Metabolism*, **54**, 711.

Boyden, T., Pamenter, R., Stanforth, P., Rotkis, T., & Wilmore, J. (1983). Sex steroids and endurance running in women. *Fertility and Sterility*, **39**, 629.

Brisson, G.R., Volle, M.A., DeCarufel, D., Desharnis, M., & Tanaka, M. (1980). Exercise-induced dissociation of the blood prolactin response in young women according to their sports habits. *Hormone and Metabolic Research*, **12**, 201.

Dale, E., Gerlach, D.H., & Wilhite, A.L. (1979). Menstrual dysfunction in distance runners. *Obstetrics and Gynecology*, **54**, 47.

Dale, E., Gerlach, D.H., Martin, D.E., & Alexander, C.R. (1979). Physical fitness profiles and reproductive physiology of the female distance runner. *The Physician and Sportsmedicine*, **7**, 83.

Erdelyi, G.J. (1962). Gynecological survey of female athletes: AMA Proceedings of the Second National Conference on the Medical Aspects of Sports, November 1960. *Journal of Sports Medicine*, **2**, 174.

Erdelyi, G.J. (1976). Effects of exercise on the menstrual cycle. *The Physician and Sportsmedicine*, **4**, 79.

Eriksson, B.O., Engstrom, L., Karlberg, P., Lundin, A., Saltin, B., & Thoren, C. (1978). Long-term effect of previous swim training in girls: A 10-year follow-up on the "Girl Swimmers." *Acta Paediatrica Scandinavica*, **67**, 85.

Feicht, C.B., Johnson, T.S., Martin, B.J., Sparkes, K.E., & Wagner, W.W. (1978). Secondary amenorrhea in athletes. *Lancet*, **2**, 1145.

Frisch, R.E., & McArthur, J.W. (1974). Menstrual cycles: Fatness as a determinant of minimum weight for height necessary for their maintenance or onset. *Science*, **185**, 949.

Frisch, R.E., Wyshak, G., & Vincent, L. (1980). Delayed menarche and amenorrhea in ballet dancers. *New England Journal of Medicine*, **303**, 17.

Frisch, R.E., Gotz-Welbergen, A., McArthur, J.W., Albright, T., Witschi, J., Bullen, B., Birnholz, J., Reed, R., & Hermann, H. (1981). Delayed menarche and amenorrhea of college athletes in relation to age of onset of training. *Journal of the American Medical Association, 246,* 1559.

Gonzalez, E.R. (1982). Premature bone loss found in some nonmenstruating sports women. *Journal of the American Medical Association, 248,* 513.

Grunby, P. (1981). Increasing numbers of physical changes found in nation's runners (Medical News). *Journal of the American Medical Association, 245,* 547.

Harris, D.V. (1978). Secondary amenorrhea linked to stress. *The Physician and Sportsmedicine, 6,* 24.

Hunter, L. (1980, June). The female athlete. *Resident and Staff Physician,* pp. 68-79.

Jurkowski, J.E., Jones, N.L., Walker, W.C., Younglai, E.V., & Sutton, J.R. (1978). Ovarian hormonal responses to exercise. *Journal of Applied Physiology, 44,* 109.

Malina, R.M., Spirduso, W., Tate, C., & Baylor, A.M. (1978). Age at menarche and selected menstrual characteristics in athletes at different competitive levels and in different sports. *Medicine and Science in Sports, 10,* 218.

Rougier, G., & Linquette, Y. (1962). Menstruation and physical exercise. *Presse Medicate, 79,* 1921.

Schlechte, J., Sherman, B., & Martin, R. (1983). Bone density in amenorrheic women with and without hyperprolactinemia. *Journal of Clinical Endocrinology and Metabolism, 56,* 1120.

Schwartz, B., Cumming, D., Riordan, E., Selye, M., Yen, S.S.C., & Rebar, R.W. (1981). Exercise-associated amenorrhea: A distinct entity? *American Journal of Obstetrics and Gynecology, 141,* 662.

Shangold, M., Freeman, R., Thysen, B., & Gatz, M. (1979). The relationship between long-distance running, plasmic progesterone and luteal phase length. *Fertility and Sterility, 31,* 130.

Shangold, M. (1980). Sports and menstrual function. *The Physician and Sportsmedicine, 8,* 66.

Shangold, M., Gatz, M.L., & Thysen, B. (1981). Acute effects of exercise on plasma concentrations of prolactin and testosterone in recreational women runners. *Fertility and Sterility, 35,* 699.

Speroff, L., & Redwine, D.B. (1980). Exercise and menstrual function. *The Physician and Sportsmedicine, 8,* 42.

Speroff, L. (1982). Moderator, symposium on impact of exercise on menstruation and reproduction. *Contemporary OB/GYN, 19*, 54-78.

Stager, J.M., Ritchie-Flanagan, B., & Robertshaw, D. (1984, January). Reversibility of amenorrhea in athletes [Letter to the editor]. *New England Journal of Medicine*, p. 51.

Warren, M.P. (1980). The effects of exercise on pubertal progression and reproductive function in girls. *Journal of Clinical Endocrinology and Metabolism, 51*, 1150.

Wentz, A.C. (1980). Body weight and amenorrhea. *Obstetrics and Gynecology, 56*, 482.

Zhanel, K. (1971). Fencing in relation to menstrual cycle and gestation. *Journal of Sports and Physical Fitness, 11*, 120.

Reactions to Elizabeth Baker's Presentation

Reactor: Leonard Calabrese

We should be thinking about some of the problems that we face in investigation of not only the epidemiology, the pathophysiology, and the sequelae of menstrual abnormalities but also potential treatments. At what point in training do menstrual abnormalities in a woman relate to her physical activity? Running a mile a day? One dance class a week? Is it when you double those numbers, triple them, or quadruple them? There are so many variables involved with the female with menstrual dysfunction who is physically active that univariate testing becomes almost impossible to interpret. Age of onset of training is controversial. The work of Frisch and colleagues in college-age runners suggests that early onset of training before menses is very significant. Our work in club-level gymnasts and elite dancers suggests just the opposite—that serious training before or after menarche really has no bearing on the menstrual cycle. Body weight and body fat are two different factors that are very closely related. The number of miles run per week has been suggested as a factor, but there are many other things going on at the same time. The person who runs more is burning up more calories. Studies have shown that women who run longer distances per week have lower body weight and usually lower body fat. Dr. Baker's preliminary observations on the amenorrheic runners who are injured more than runners with normal menses can be interpreted as meaning people who run more are probably more prone to overuse injury. Those injuries will have to be scrutinized to finally interpret those data.

These data (unnamed on the slide but well referenced) on a variety of female athletes show that club-level gymnasts and professional ballet dancers have delayed menarche just as elite runners do. These are all very demanding physical activities, but as sporting activities they are quite different. In gymnasts and professional ballet dancers, menarche is significantly delayed, the onset of secondary amenorrhea is very high (33 and 40% in these two groups), and the number of irregular cycles is as high as in any groups reported. How does this compare to the running females? Gymnasts and ballet dancers share low percent body fat with runners. Perhaps this is the unifying hypothesis. On the other hand, the mechanism of their body fat production is markedly different, and we may just be biasing our view if we look at the incidence of menstrual problems as being solely a function of this. If we now look at the VO_2max, going from our elite runners to sedentary women, we can see some very striking differences. Ballet and gymnastics, particularly at the club level, and professional dancing, are not aerobic exercises. The works of Kirkendall and Cohen have shown quite conclusively that this is nonendurance training, very demanding, very punishing, but not an aerobic type of exercise because of the nature of dance and gymnastics. So we have two groups of female athletes with a very, very high incidence of menstrual abnormalities, both low in body fat, but with some major differences in their training.

The logical question is why are they so lean even though they are not engaged predominantly in aerobic activities? What about the nutritional aspects of athletics? Along with stress, the contribution of nutrition to these problems is a poorly studied area. Dr. Dale and others have shown that long distance female runners take in more than the RDA for calories and most vital nutrients. From our study group, 76% of our ballet dancers were taking in less than 85% of the RDA for calories, 40% were taking in less than 66% of the RDA, and 25% were taking in less than 50% of the RDA. If you are only taking in 50 to 60% of the RDA, you had better have a very well-defined and planned diet to obtain essential nutrients. The data show that these women do not. The mineral intakes of this group are frightening. In our data, there was no correlation whatsoever between body fat and any combination of menstrual abnormalities.

Discussion

Robert Marcus: Several of us have agreed that a number of different institutions have derived some rather startling data about calorie intake. The older idea that female runners are taking in more calories is not right. We have tried as compulsively as we can to do nutrient intake analysis and we found rather severe calorie deficits. To my knowledge, there is no such thing as an RDA for calories. When you talk about RDAs for calories, where are you getting the numbers?

Dr. Calabrese: The National Research Council has established age-related RDAs for calories for the "sedentary female" of average body weight. These are very conservative and very rough.

Robert Marcus: I think it is much more important to report calorie data quantitatively because the RDA number is a fantasy number.

Dr. Calabrese: I do this to be a provocateur. What is important is that we observed a group of females taking in less than 600 calories a day and dancing 40 hours a week. There is a direct relationship between caloric density and nutritional density, and you are much more prone to take in adequate nutritional elements if you are taking in a lot of calories than if you are taking in only a few calories.

Michelle Warren: Before you make conclusions about training and the age of menarche, I think it is important to compare girls of similar physique. Data indicate that the hypothalamic amenorrhea that you are interested in is very definitely related to body weight. Body fat is undoubtedly important in some way and probably influences neural interrelationships. It is very hard to compare one study to another because of the different methods used in measuring body fat and the errors inherent in the method. In our longitudinal study on ballet and professional dancers, the onset of pubertal development is so dramatic when training stops that there is a type of "catch-up." Normal pubertal development in women takes up to 2 years from the first state to the last. These kids can go through all four or five states in 4 months. So, longitudinal studies are very important.

Joan Ullyot: What has bothered me, particularly about the running studies, is that so many researchers who may not be familiar with runners rely on mileage as a means of determining how stressful their running is. Much more important than the mileage, in my experience, is the quality of the work. You should expect information on the Stanford cross-country team, which has very intense interval speed work, to be different from data on a woman who runs 80 miles a week but all at 10 minutes a mile. I think this is another variable we really have to look at in these studies.

Jerilynn Prior: Some of us who like to run or play a particular sport have crossed over a frontier from having to be the perfect female who is passive and sedentary to wanting to be a perfect female who is athletic as well as feminine. The press might look at some of the available information on women in athletics, find something "dangerous," and say, "See, you should not be doing that!" We do not want to find bad, awful things but we do want to find out what's going on. We have to be honest with our patients, our colleagues, our friends, and ourselves about any possible danger, but we do not want to find anything wrong. The history of women in sport has been clouded by reluctance to face facts. Women have been accepted in the marathon. Women are known to be good athletes. We now can say, "Look, in women we have a unique situation, a biological system that is different from the one we've usually looked at in athletics. Let's find out how this unique biological system, especially the reproductive system, responds to athletic activity."

2

The Menstrual Cycle and Athletic Performance

Jeanne Brooks-Gunn
Educational Testing Service
Janine Gargiulo
University of Virginia
Michelle P. Warren
St. Luke's-Roosevelt Hospital Center

Many athletes believe that menstruation negatively affects their performance, just as many women believe that motoric and cognitive performance is impaired during the perimenstruum. From one third to one half of all women believe that their performance is impaired by menstruation, even though decrements are, for the most part, nonexistent. In two comprehensive reviews (Sommer, 1973, 1983), few if any consistent menstrual-related performance decrements were found in studies of nonathletic women.

Given the large literature on possible menstrual-related performance effects, it is somewhat surprising that little information exists on possible links between cycle phase and athletes' performance. Anecdotal accounts suggest that some women have recorded their best performances and won major competitions during their menses (Delaney, Lupton, & Toth, 1976; Ryan, 1975). At the same time, some elite athletes have reported to the press that they are negatively affected by menstruation. Up to one third of all athletes subscribe to this belief. For example, one third of a sample of 1960 Olympic participants felt menstruation adversely affected their performance (Zaharieva, 1965).

In this chapter, we will review what is known about cycle phase effects on athletic performance. In addition, factors which may influence cycle phase-

The research reported in this chapter was supported by an IBM Fellowship awarded to the second author and grants from the W.T. Grant Foundation and the National Institutes of Health. Rosemary Deibler is to be thanked for help with manuscript preparation.

performance relationships will be reviewed. Socialization practices, different contexts, cultural beliefs, and biological processes will be considered as possible factors. Finally, limitations of our current knowledge will be discussed, with recommendations for future research on possible cycle phase-performance links.

Cycle-Related Performance Effects

Early Studies

At least five studies on athletic performance and cycle phase were performed prior to 1970 on the following groups of women: (a) 1,435 women, with 553 who were engaged in regular intensive exercise, 309 who exercised 2 to 4 hours weekly, and 573 who did not exercise (Rougier & Linquette, 1962); (b) an unspecified number of athletes participating in the 1930 Track and Field Championships in Prague (Kral & Markalous, 1937); (c) 104 Finnish sportswomen (Ingman, 1952); (d) 66 sportswomen participating in the Tokyo Olympics (Zaharieva, 1965); and (e) 557 athletes, with no specifics given (Erdelyi, 1962).

In the earliest study, Kral and Markalous (1937) found performance decrements during menses for 8% of the participants in the 1930 Track and Field Championships, performance enhancements for 29%, and no performance effect for 63%. In the study of Finnish sportswomen (Ingman, 1952), 19% reported best performances during menses, 38% reported poorest performance during menses, and 43% reported no change. Interestingly, 24% did not ordinarily compete during menses due to pain and/or fatigue. These women may account for a large proportion of those reporting poor menstrual performances. In their questionnaire survey of athletes, Rougier and Linquette (1962) reported that 59% suffer a decrease in performance and an increase in symptoms premenstrually, and an additional 11% reported a decrease in speed and strength premenstrually, even though they reported no cycle-related symptoms. Zaharieva (1965) reported that 37% of his sample from the Tokyo Olympics showed no performance decrements, 28% showed a variation in performance (although it was not specified in which direction the variation occurred), and 17% showed a performance decrement. In all four of these studies, performance seems to have been measured by self-reports; therefore, these findings are likely to be confounded with beliefs about performance decrements.

In the final study (Erdelyi, 1962), 42% to 48% of over 500 athletes showed no cycle phase effects, 31% exhibited performance decrements, and 13% to 15% showed performance enhancements during menstruation. Best performances were reported in the postmenstrual phase. In addition, the author reported that "poor performances can be found in an overwhelming majority in the premenstruum and the first two days of the menstrual period, while during the latter days of the period the sports performance may be much better than during the first days of the period." Finally, the incidence of cycle-related performance decrements varies as a function of type of sport. One half of the tennis players and rowers exhibited extremely poor menstrual performance; fewer athletes participating in ball games, swimming, and gymnastics exhibited decrements, and some even exhibited menstrual cycle enhancements. The amount of effort exerted by the athlete and the length of time over which this effort must be exerted are the two possible explanations offered in the study for these differential effects. It was hypothesized that tennis players and rowers would exert a great deal of effort for a long period of time whereas ball players, swimmers, and gymnasts would exert an effort for a shorter time period. Put another way, performance during menstruation may be poor in sports where endurance is involved, while in sports where short bursts of activity are essential, performance may be enhanced during menses. No test of this hypothesis has been made, however, nor have possible mechanisms underlying such an effect been studied.

In summary, 40% to 60% of all athletes in these studies do not seem to show cycle-related performance alterations, and 15% to 30% exhibit their worst performance in the menstrual and/or premenstrual phase (early studies often did not differentiate between these phases). Therefore, the limited evidence to date suggests that not all athletes exhibit performance changes linked to cycle phases. For some women in certain sports, performance may be enhanced during menstruation.

Recent Studies

To our knowledge only one study (Brooks-Gunn, Gargiulo, & Warren, in press) has been recently conducted to examine possible performance decrements associated with the perimenstruum. Six adolescent girls who were members of a competitive swim team and who were practicing 4 to 5 hours daily were followed for 3 months. Their coach timed each girl's performance twice a week for 10 weeks during normally scheduled practices. Best performance in the 100-yd freestyle and 100-yd best event (other than freestyle) was assessed. The coach was blind as to the girls' cycle phase. In addition, girls were contacted weekly thereafter to record their menstrual days.

Average performance times were calculated for (a) the entire cycle, (b) the postmenstrual phase (the 10 days after menstruation ceased), (c) the premenstrual phase (the 4 days prior to the onset of menstruation), and (d) the menstrual phase (the duration of the menstrual flow). In the 100-yd freestyle, premenstrual performance was .96 s slower and menstrual performance was .82 s faster than the average time. Findings were similar for best event; premenstrual performance was 1.32 s slower and menstrual performance was

.70 s faster than the average. These differences were seen in all 4 subjects who menstruated during the study. In addition, the fastest time across the 18 performance time trials for 3 of the 4 subjects was recorded during the menstrual phase; the slowest time for 2 of the 4 subjects occurred in the premenstrual phase. Possible explanations of the menstrual enhancement effect include the fluid reduction associated with menstruation, self-expectancies, thermoregulation, and the absence of dysmenorrhea. All of these will be discussed in the following section.

Mediators of Cycle-Related Performance Effects

Self-Expectancies

The idea that a person's behavior is affected by his or her expectations regarding that behavior has received considerable attention in the social psychology literature. For example, achievement-related outcomes have been shown to be influenced by one's expectations concerning such outcomes (Archibald, 1974). The placebo effect illustrates a similar phenomenon. In addition, people's behavior also conforms to the expectations and treatment of others. The most well-known example is found in Rosenthal and Jacobson's *Pygmalion in the Classroom* (1968). In this study, teachers were told that a randomly selected group of students in their classroom would make great intellectual gains in the school year; students who were expected to "bloom" intellectually made greater gains during the school year than those who were not expected to do so.

The self-fulfilling prophecy that expectations for behavior influence its occurrence has been applied in interpreting the menstruation literature. It has been hypothesized that expectancies concerning cycle-related debilitation would lead to reports of symptoms. Support for a self-fulfilling prophecy is found in a longitudinal study (Brooks-Gunn & Ruble, 1982, 1983) of 120 premenarcheal girls who were reinterviewed 2 and 9 months after menarche. Specifically, premenarcheal girls who expected to experience more severe menstrual symptoms actually reported more severe symptoms after the onset of menarche. These findings could not be accounted for by differences in maternal symptoms. The theory underlying this assumes that if there is a genetic predisposition for menstrual symptomatology, premenarcheal girls' expectations could be influenced by their mothers' experiences, which in turn could be related to the daughters' actual symptomatology; however, links between maternal and daughter symptomatology were not found. With regard to actual performance rather than the report of symptoms, no evidence exists that expectations about performance are related to actual performance. For example, being hesitant about reaching top performance during menstruation was not related to actually reaching top performance (Zaharieva, 1965).

Another way to test the hypothesis that menstrual-related expectations lead to behavior changes is to vary experimentally expectations regarding changes associated with the menstrual cycle and then to observe behavioral effects. In one such study (Baird, 1975), women were told that women in the menstrual phase (as opposed to the intermenstrual phase) typically performed either better (because of higher levels of arousal) or worse (because of difficulties concentrating) on particular kinds of tasks. The women were then asked to do the tasks (digit symbol substitution and bicycling) either during their intermenstrual or menstrual phases. Contrary to predictions, no differences in performance across expectation conditions nor cycle phases were found. Similar findings are reported by Altenhouse (1978) and Munchel (1976). Thus, although there are strong beliefs about menstrual-related performance effects, few effects are found (Ruble & Brooks-Gunn, 1979). Beliefs concerning negative affect changes rather than beliefs about performance are more likely to result in a self-fulfilling prophecy, as was found in the longitudinal study of adolescent girls reported earlier.

Cultural Restrictions and Menstruation

The menstrual flow is almost universally perceived as negative and is considered unclean and perhaps even dangerous in many societies, even when medical information is given to the contrary (Brooks-Gunn, in press; Delaney, Lupton, & Toth, 1976). In addition, restrictions on sexuality, food preparation, personal habits, and social activities are common cross-culturally (Paige, 1974). In our culture, up to one quarter of all women restrict physical and social activities (bathing, sports participation) during menses (Paige, 1974). Do such culturally sanctioned restrictions affect athletes' training regimes? Twenty years ago, 12% of Olympic athletes never trained during their menses, 54% trained irregularly or sometimes, and 34% always trained (Zaharieva, 1965). Although no data exist, it is expected that virtually all athletes compete during menses today, although training regimes may vary.

Swimmers may be most likely not to train or compete during menses due to the belief that swimming in cold water is unhealthy and that swimming without internal protection is unsanitary. Of the swimmers in the 1964 Olympics, 33% did not train during menses (as opposed to 12% of other competitors). This finding may in part be explained by the fact that tampon use was not accepted for unmarried women and for adolescents at that time. Today, over 70% of American girls 16 years and older use tampons. However, fewer younger adolescents use them; 25% of 12- and 13-year-olds and 40% of 14-year-olds report using tampons (Brooks-Gunn & Ruble, 1982). Thus, young swimmers may be more likely to alter their training schedules than older swimmers. One quarter of American women believe in restricting sports, particularly swimming, and bathing during menstruation (Paige, 1974).

Perceptual-Motor Performance

Although no menstrual decrements are found for the majority of cognitive, perceptual, and motoric skills, there are three for which cycle-related differences have been reported. First, complex reaction time (a choice among stimulus or response must be made prior to responding) may be slower premenstrually than at other times during the month (Gamberale, Strindberg, & Wahlberg, 1975; Hunter, Schraer, Landers, Buskirk, & Harris, 1979; Landauer, 1974). However, an equal number of studies (Sommer, 1983) have found no cycle phase effects for complex reaction time.

Second, arm-hand steadiness may be better at midcycle than at other times of the month (Zimmerman & Parlee, 1973). In a study of basketball and volleyball players, stationary hand steadiness was adversely affected in the premenstruum (Wearing, Yuhosz, Campbell, & Love, 1972).

Third, visual discrimination may be less sensitive premenstrually, although the effects are measure-specific and small. For example, when the measure was speed of reaction to a constant light that begins to flicker, 16 subjects showed the fastest times in the luteal phase, when progesterone and estradiol were highest. In addition, a positive correlation between progesterone and estradiol and speed of reaction time was found (Wuttke et al., 1976). In another study (Ward, Stone, & Sandman, 1978) measuring hormonal levels, 12 women were asked to report the presence or absence of a dot, thought to be a measure of visual sensitivity. Visual accuracy was highest during the menstrual phase; in addition, estradiol levels and percentage of correct detection scores were found to be related. Several studies (Sommer, 1983) have examined fine temporal discriminations in what is called the two flash-fusion threshold paradigm. This is the point at which a subject reports two successive light flashes as one. Decreased sensitivity premenstrually was found in some but not all studies. Visual discrimination is usually important in many sports.

Physical Fitness

Another possibility is that women have less endurance during the premenstruum. Of the few studies conducted, one found no differences in ISK mile and 600-yd run (Doolittle & Engebretsen, 1972). In another (Wearing et al., 1972), hip strength flexion and extension did not vary as a function of cycle phase. Thus, little evidence for fitness differences across cycle phases exists.

Menstrual Symptoms

Performance decrements may be due in part to the existence of specific menstrual symptoms such as dysmenorrhea, water retention, or negative affect. However, before focusing on particular symptom clusters, it is important to discuss the limitations of self-report data. Symptoms are usually assessed by asking women to judge the severity of symptoms they experience during different cycle phases based on a series of scales. When asked directly about menstrual-related symptoms in this way, women typically report that they experience significantly more negative symptoms during the premenstrual and menstrual phases than at other times of the month. These self-reports provide the major data base for statements concerning the prevalence and extent of cyclic fluctuations. Research, however, has shown that the information obtained from self-reports is systematically biased by women's awareness that the purpose of the questionnaire is to study menstrual symptoms and by her perception of what phase of the cycle (premenstrual, menstrual, or other) she is in. For example, many cyclic fluctuations tend to be found only when women are asked to report retrospectively about their typical experience. Retrospective reports seem to highlight the association between phase of the cycle and symptoms (Ruble & Brooks-Gunn, 1979). However, prospective reports (e.g., daily ratings of current experience of symptoms) often fail to show cyclic fluctuations, especially when the woman is unaware of the nature of the study (Englander-Golden, Whitmore, & Dienstbier, 1978).

Thus, one must question the validity of self-report data unless it is prospective and an attempt is made to "blind" the subject as to the nature of the study. Reviewing studies that meet these criteria, Ruble and Brooks-Gunn (1979) found that only two of the 8 symptom clusters typically studied exhibited consistent phase differences; these are pain and water retention. More recent studies support this finding (Ruble & Brooks-Gunn, 1984). Differences are found for a third symptom cluster, premenstrual negative affect, in about one half of all well-designed prospective studies. Findings on each of these symptom clusters will be briefly reviewed as they relate to athletic performance.

Dysmenorrhea   *Dysmenorrhea*, or menstrual abdominal pain, is reported by 60% to 75% of all adult women; it increases with chronologic and gynecologic age. In two large Finnish studies (Widholm, 1979; Widholm & Kantero, 1971), 40% of those in the first postmenarcheal year, 50% in the second, and 65% in the third reported dysmenorrhea. Severity increased with gynecologic and chronologic age in a large sample of New Jersey adolescents and college students (Brooks-Gunn & Ruble, 1983). However, it must be stressed that the vast majority (75% to 80%) of those reporting dysmenorrhea rate it as mild, not severe (Ruble & Brooks-Gunn, 1979; Widholm, 1979).

Dysmenorrhea is the only menstrual symptom for which specific biological causes have been identified. Prostaglandins released from the endometrium are a major cause of dysmenorrhea, as demonstrated by clinical trials using prostaglandin synthesis inhibitors as dysmenorrhea treatment (Chan, Dawood, & Fuchs, 1981; Ylikorkala & Dawood, 1978). Chan (1983) examined levels of prostaglandins and menstrual blood in dysmenorrheic and nondysmenorrheic women, finding that the majority (but not all) of dysmenorrheic women have high levels of menstrual prostaglandins. Dysmenorrhea also may be reduced through the use of oral contraceptives; when ovulation is inhibited, hypoplasia of the endometrium may occur, reducing the ability of the endometrium to produce prostaglandins.

Specific links between prostaglandins and dysmenorrhea have been demonstrated elegantly. However, there are some questions which remain. For example, it is not clear why some women have higher levels of prostaglandins than others, why not all women with dysmenorrhea exhibit high levels of prostaglandins, why within-subject variation occurs over cycles and time, or why self-reports of dysmenorrhea may differ for women with similar prostaglandin output. Biological predispositions to higher levels of prostaglandins, cyclic variations in neuroendocrine functioning, differences in pain threshold, and psychological processes such as symptom denial may contribute to these as yet unresolved issues.

Much of our information about dysmenorrhea in athletes is anecdotal because few investigators have asked athletes to chart symptoms over time. In the early study by Erdelyi (1962), menstrual "disorders" including dysmenorrhea, oligomenorrhea, amenorrhea, and polymenorrhea are reported in 18% of those athletes under 17 and in 7% of those athletes over 18. Unfortunately, no figures are given for dysmenorrhea separately.

In a large retrospective study (Timonen & Procopé, 1971) of 748 college students, some of whom were athletes, the presence or absence of menstrual pain (rather than severity or frequency) was assessed. The athletes reported less menstrual and premenstrual pain and took analgesics less frequently than the nonathletes. Dale, Gerlach, and Wilhite (1979) also reported fewer cramps in runners than in controls. And in our small sample, none of the swimmers reported dysmenorrhea during the premenstrual or menstrual phase of the cycle (Brooks-Gunn, Gargiulo, & Warren, in press).

The lower incidence and/or severity of dysmenorrhea in athletes could be due to lower levels of prostaglandins which in turn could be due to a higher number of anovulatory cycles or altered endocrine patterns (less step LH surge, short luteal phase, lower levels of estradiol and/or progesterone). Alternatively, athletes may have higher pain thresholds or may be more likely to deny the effects of pain, given their training experiences. In our swimmer study, the most frequently mentioned symptom across all cycle phases was sore muscles (especially arm muscles); however, the swimmers did not believe that this almost constant soreness affected their performance. Instead, it was seen as an inevitable consequence of training.

Water Retention The triad of fluid retention, sore or tender breasts, and enlarged breasts also has been verified in the majority of adequately controlled prospective studies. Unlike dysmenorrhea, the etiology is not well understood, and a number of mechanisms have been proposed to account for this symptom cluster. In one of the few studies attempting to directly study the links between water retention and etiology, Janowsky, Davis, and Berens (1972) asked 11 women to rate symptoms of severity daily for several cycles; morning weights were taken and urine also was collected in order to obtain potassium-sodium ratios thought to be a measure of fluid retention. Actual weight and potassium-sodium ratios increased and decreased in synchrony over the cycle period. Top weight was obtained 1 to 4 days prior to menses and weight loss occurred on the first day of menses. Potassium-sodium ratios peaked 3 days before menstruation and decreased on the first day of menses. An earlier study (Abramson & Torghele, 1961) actually charted daily changes in weight and self-reported feelings of bloatedness and other symptoms. In accord with the Janowsky study, weight was higher premenstrually, beginning to drop on the day prior to menses, and continuing to drop over the first 2 days of menses. In general, symptoms decreased with weight loss, although a separate analysis by symptom cluster was not performed.

In our study, reported severity of water retention was highest premenstrually and lowest menstrually, in line with the two studies just cited. Timonen and Procopé (1971) also did not find fewer cases of water retention in university athletes than in nonathletes. Thus, the few studies to date are consistent in reporting that athletes, while being less likely to experience dysmenorrhea, are equally likely to experience premenstrual water retention when compared to nonathletes.

Premenstrual Tension Approximately one half of all prospective daily symptom report studies find premenstrual increases in negative affect (Ruble & Brooks-Gunn, 1979; Sommer, 1983).[1] More recently, prospective studies (e.g., Abplanalp, Donnelly, & Rose, 1979) have not found negative changes during the premenstruum. However, 50% to 60% of all women, including adolescents, report retrospectively that they experience negative affect premenstrually (Brooks-Gunn & Ruble, 1983; Widholm, 1979). No increases were found as a function of gynecological or chronological age in these two studies. Given the lack of increase with gynecological age and the mixed

---

[1]It is critical to distinguish between premenstrual tension and the premenstrual syndrome (PMS). A syndrome has specific diagnostic criteria. The literature is unclear as to whether a premenstrual syndrome exists and as to the number of women affected, if it does exist. For example, in one study of 130 women responding to an advertisement for women with severe PMS, only 8, or 5%, met the specific diagnostic criteria (Hoskett & Abplanalp, 1983). It is quite likely that no more than 1/2 of 1% of all women would meet the diagnostic criteria for PMS. Another problem has to do with the etiology of PMS. No definitive evidence exists for the physiological basis of PMS, in spite of the large number of theories advanced. In a similar vein, placebos are as effective as any of the treatments attempted to date, as summarized in a recent conference on PMS sponsored by NSF. At the same time, popular beliefs concerning the prevalence of severe PMS continue or have even increased in the last few years (Parlee, in press).

results of prospective studies, it is likely that cultural beliefs and socialization influence the report of negative affect.

The belief in premenstrual negative affect may have indirect effects on other symptom reports. For example, the association of pain with menstruation may itself result in emotional changes such as irritability. As another example, certain social contexts or experiences may influence cultural beliefs and/or physiological states. We know that within certain religious and ethnic groups, it is considered inappropriate to discuss menarche (Abel & Joffe, 1950). We also know that girls who are unprepared for menarche report the experience to be distressing and the symptoms to be more severe (Ruble & Brooks-Gunn, 1982). Associations between menstruation and distress may continue, as girls are more likely to label internal states as cycle induced. They also may be anxious around the time of menstruation, given their initial negative experience and expectations for continuing negative experiences, which in turn may influence hormonal secretions or sensitivity to hormonal change. As an example, possible interactions between factors contributing to self reports of premenstrual negative affect are illustrated in Figure 1.

Figure 1

An example of interactions between factors contributing to premenstrual negative affect.

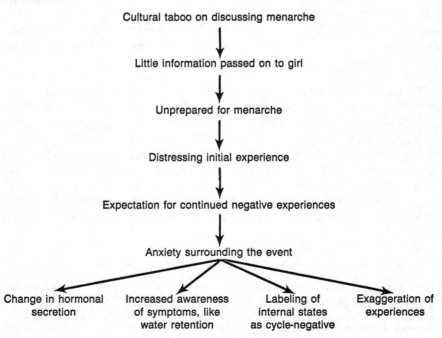

To return to athletes' symptom reports, athletes report less negative affect than nonathletes (Timonen & Procopé, 1971) and no negative affect in our small sample of adolescent swimmers (Brooks-Gunn et al., 1984). Whether these differences are biologically, culturally, or socially induced is not known.

Other Cycle Characteristics

Cycle-phase performance effects may be mediated in part by other cycle characteristics, either through biological or psychological mechanisms. Three such menstrual characteristics are anovulatory cycles, short luteal phases, and intensity of menses. As many of the chapters in this volume illustrate, athletes have a disproportionately large number of anovulatory cycles, even after controlling for gynecological age. In addition, short luteal phases may be common even in biphasic cycles (Bonen, Belcastro, Ling, & Simpson, 1981). In cycles with relatively low levels of estradiol and progesterone, or an inadequate LH surge midcycle, dysmenorrhea is less likely to occur, as inferred from the findings on oral contraceptives. In fact, athletes are less likely to report dysmenorrhea, perhaps due to low levels of prostaglandins. In addition, other symptoms may be less likely to occur in athletes premenstrually, most specifically fluid retention and sore breasts. However, this possibility has not been verified by the few relevant studies. Indeed, we suspect that the menstrual performance enhancement reported in our study (Brooks-Gunn, Gargiulo, & Warren, in press) is due to reduced water retention as well as the feelings of energy that occurred during the menstrual phase.

Intensity of menstrual flow may be reduced in athletes due to hypoplasia of the endometrium. In nonathletes, length of the menstrual flow is positively related to self-reported symptomatology, perceptions of menstrual debilitation, and performance expectations, as reported in samples of college women (Brooks-Gunn, in press; Paige, 1974). Because athletes may experience lighter and/or shorter flows, they may perceive menstruation as being less debilitating than nonathletes. In brief, cycle characteristics may alter symptom experiences or reports, which in turn influence cycle-related performance.

Recommendations for Research

In general, the paucity of research on the effects of cycle phase upon performance is startling, especially given the interest in menstruation and the female athlete, as evidenced by the excellent contributions found in this volume. Perhaps research has not been conducted because beliefs in cycle-related performance decrements are so pervasive. Reliance on retrospective self-reports in the early studies reflects the cultural belief in impairment during menses.

Our intriguing and perhaps even provocative finding (Brooks-Gunn, Gargiulo, & Warren, in press) that performance is best during the menstrual phase and worst during the premenstrual phase hopefully will result in other studies. It is critical that the participants and coaches in such studies be "blind" to the investigators' hypotheses and, if possible, interest in cycle phase effects. Studies could be presented as an investigation of changes in performance over time or with competition.

Of particular interest are possible individual variations in cycle phase performance effects. Whether differences are studied across women or across cycles in individuals, such comparisons allow for a better understanding of the consistency of effects and the possible contribution of various factors to the phenomenon. For example, if dysmenorrhea is implicated, then women with and without this symptom may be compared with regard to cycle phase effects. As another example, if performance decrements or enhancements appear evident only in ovulatory or biphasic cycles, studies might include basal body temperature (BBT) assessments in addition to performance measurements. Finally, the question of fluid retention and reduction as mediators of performance could be studied by measuring daily weight changes.

Several investigators have suggested that the menstrual cycle will affect performance differently as a function of the sport studied. Therefore, studies could compare athletes in different sports; sports could be chosen that vary on dimensions involving energy expended, endurance, agility, muscles required, and so on.

In summary, performance may vary as a function of cycle phase, at least for some athletes, in some cycles, and in some sports. Given the importance of such variations in high-level competition and the potential for impact of beliefs upon performance, we urge our colleagues to broaden their prospective studies to include performance measures, when possible.

References

Abel, T., & Joffe, N.F. (1950). Cultural background of female puberty. *American Journal of Psychotherapy*, **4**, 90-93.

Abplanalp, J.M., Donnelly, A.F., & Rose, R.M. (1979). Psychoendocrinology of the menstrual cycle: I. Enjoyment of daily activities and moods. *Psychosomatic Medicine*, **41**, 587-604.

Abramson, M., & Torghele, J.R. (1961). *American Journal of Obstetrics and Gynecology*, **81**, 223.

Altenhouse, A.L. (1978). *The effect of expectancy for change on performance during the menstrual cycle.* Unpublished doctoral dissertation, Rutgers University, New Brunswick, NJ.

Archibald, W.P. (1974). Alternative explanations for self-fulfilling prophecy. *Psychological Bulletin,* **81,** 74-84.

Baird, B.S. (1975). *An experimental study of the effects of menstrual cycle related expectancies on performance and attributions.* Unpublished senior thesis, Princeton University, Princeton, NJ.

Bonen, A., Belcastro, A.N., Ling, W.Y., & Simpson, A.A. (1981). Profiles of selected hormones during menstrual cycles of teenage athletes. *Journal of Applied Physiological Respiratory Environmental Exercise Physiology,* **50**(3), 545-551.

Brooks-Gunn, J. (in press). The salience and timing of the menstrual flow. *Psychosomatic Medicine.*

Brooks-Gunn, J., Gargiulo, J., & Warren, M.P. (in press). The effect of cycle phase upon adolescent swimmers' performance. *The Physician and Sportsmedicine.*

Brooks-Gunn, J., & Ruble, D.N. (1983). The experience of menarche from a developmental perspective. In J. Brooks-Gunn and A.C. Petersen (Eds.), *Girls at puberty: Biological and psychosocial perspectives* (pp. 155-177). New York: Plenum Press.

Brooks-Gunn, J., & Ruble, D.N. (1982). Psychological determinants of menstrual product use in adolescent females. *Annals of Internal Medicine,* **96**(6), 962-965.

Chan, W.Y. (1983). Prostaglandins in primary dysmenorrhea: Basis for the new therapy. In S. Golub (Ed.), *Menarche* (pp. 243-249). Lexington, MA: Lexington Books.

Chan, W.Y., Dawood, M.Y., & Fuchs, F. (1981). Prostaglandins in primary dysmenorrhea comparison of prophylactic and nonprophylactic treatment with ibuprofen and use of oral contraceptives. *American Journal of Medicine,* **70,** 535-541.

Dale, E., Gerlach, D., & Wilhite, A. (1979). Menstrual dysfunction in distance runners. *Obstetrics and Gynecology,* **54**(1), 47-53.

Delany, J., Lupton, J.J., & Toth, E. (1976). *The curse: A cultural history of menstruation.* New York: Dutton.

Doolittle, T.L., & Engebretsen, J. (1972). Performance variations during the menstrual cycle. *Journal of Sports Medicine and Physical Fitness,* **12**(5), 54-58.

Englander-Golden, P., Whitmore, M.R., & Dienstbier, R.A. (1978). Menstrual cycle as a focus of study and self-reports of moods and behaviors. *Motivation and Emotion*, **2**, 75-86.

Erdelyi, G.J. (1962). Gynecological survey of female athletes. *Journal of Sports Medicine in Physical Fitness*, **2**, 174-179.

Gamberale, F., Strindberg, L., & Walhlberg, I. (1975). Female work capacity during the menstrual cycle: Physiological and psychological reactions. *Scandinavian Journal of Work and Environmental Health*, **1**, 120-127.

Hoskett, R.F., & Abplanalp, J.M. (1983). Premenstrual tension syndrome: Diagnostic criteria and the selection of research subjects. *Psychiatric Research*, **9**, 125.

Hunter, S., Schraer, R., Landers, D.M., Buskirk, E.R., & Harris, D.V. (1979). The effects of total estrogen concentration and menstrual-cycle phase on reaction time performance. *Ergonomics*, **22**, 263-268.

Ingman, O. (1952). Menstruation in Finnish top class sportswomen. In *Sports Medicine*—International symposium of the Medicine and Physiology of Sports and Athletes (pp. 96-98). Helsinki: Finnish Association of Sports Medicine.

Janowsky, D.S., Davis, J.M., & Berens, S.C. (1972) *Journal of the American Medical Association*, **222**(4), 417-418.

Kral, J., & Markalous, E. (1937). The influence of menstruation on sport performance. In A. Mallwitz (Ed.), *Proceedings of the Second International Congress on Sports Medicine*. Leipzig: Thieme.

Landauer, A.A. (1974). Choice decision time and the menstrual cycle. *Practitioner*, **213**, 703-706.

Munchel, M. (1976). *The effect of social and personal expectations on perceptual-motor performance during the premenstrual and midcycle phases of the menstrual cycle*. Unpublished doctoral dissertation, Indiana University.

Paige, D.E. (1974). The curse: Possible antecedents of menstrual distress. In A.A. Harrison (Ed.), *Explorations in psychology*. Monterery, CA: Brooks/Cole.

Parlee, M.B. (1984, September). *Premenstrual syndrome in the media*. Paper presented at Conference on Legal and Ethical Implications of the Biobehavioral Sciences: Premenstrual Syndrome, Philadelphia, PA.

Parlee, M.B. (in press). Media treatment of PMS. In B.F. Carter and F.E. Ginsburg (Eds.), *Legal and ethical implications of the biobehavioral sciences: Premenstrual syndrome*. New York: Plenum Press.

Rosenthal, R., & Jacobson, L. (1968). *Pygmalion in the classroom: Teacher expectation and pupils' intellectual development.* New York: Holt, Rinehart, and Winston.

Rougier, G., & Linquette, Y. (1962). Menstruation and physical exercise. *Presse Medicale,* **70,** 1921.

Ruble, D.N., & Brooks-Gunn, J. (in press). Perceptions of menstrual and premenstrual symptoms: Self definitional processes at menarche. In B.F. Carter and F.E. Ginsburg (Eds.), *Legal and ethical implications of the biobehavioral science: Premenstrual syndrome.* New York: Plenum Press.

Ruble, D.N., & Brooks-Gunn, J. (1982). The experience of menarche. *Child Development,* **53,** 1557-1566.

Ruble, D.N., & Brooks-Gunn, J. (1979). Menstrual symptoms: A social cognition analysis. *Journal of Behavioral Medicine,* **2**(2).

Ryan, A.J. (1975, January). Gynecological considerations. *JOPER,* 40-44.

Sommer, B. (1983). How does menstruation affect cognitive competence and psychophysiological response? In S. Golub (Ed.), *Lifting the curse of menstruation: A feminist appraisal of the influence of menstruation on women's lives* (pp. 53-90). New York: Haworth Press.

Sommer, B. (1973). The effect of menstruation on cognitive and perceptual-motor behavior: A review. *Psychosomatic Medicine,* **33,** 411-428.

Timonen, S., & Procopé, B.J. (1971). Premenstrual syndrome and physical exercise. *Acta Obstetrica et Gynecologica Scandinavia,* **50,** 331-337.

Ward, M.M., Stone, S.C., & Sandman, C.A. (1978). Visual perception in women during the menstrual cycle. *Physiology and Behavior,* **20,** 239-243.

Wearing, M., Yuhosz, M.D., Campbell, R., & Love, E.J. (1972). The effect of the menstrual cycle on tests of physical fitness. *Journal of Sports Medicine and Physical Fitness,* **12**(1), 38-41.

Widholm, O. (1979). Dysmenorrhea during adolescence. *Acta Obstetrica et Gynaecologica Scandinavica,* **87,** 61-66.

Widholm, O., & Kantero, R.L. (1971). Menstrual pattern of adolescent girls according to chronological and gynecological ages. *Acta Obstetrica et Gynecologica Scandinavica,* **14,** 19-29.

Wuttke, W., Arnold, P., Becker, D., Creutzfeldt, O., Langenstein, S., & Tirschy, W. (1976). Hormonal profiles and variations of the EEG and of performances in psychological tests in women with spontaneous menstrual cycles and under oral contraceptives. In T.H. Itil (Ed.), *Psychotropic action of hormones* (pp. 169-182). New York: Spectrum Publications.

Ylikorkala, O., & Dawood, M.Y. (1978). New concept in dysmenorrhea. *American Journal of Obstetrics and Gynecology*, **130**, 833-847.

Zaharieva, E. (1965). Survey of sportswomen at the Tokyo Olympics. *Journal of Sports Medicine and Physical Fitness*, **5**(4), 215-219.

Zimmerman, E., & Parlee, M.B. (1973). Behavioral changes associated with the menstrual cycle: An experimental investigation. *Journal of Applied Social Psychology*, **3**, 335-344.

3

Prevalence of Menstrual
Change in Athletes and Active Women

Judy Mahle Lutter
Melpomene Institute

What degree of menstrual change will be found in a population of athletes and active women at any given moment? This is an important question. The prevalence of menstrual change in active women has been variously documented in the past 10 years, with figures ranging from a low of 3.4% (Lutter & Cushman, 1982) to a high of 66% (Bonen & Keizer,1984). The reasons for such a wide range of findings may be enumerated as follows:

1. Definitions of menstrual cycle regularity are not uniform.
2. The methodologies used to gather and interpret information are often dissimilar.
3. The differences in age and intensity of exercise in the women studied make comparisons difficult. Athletes, particularly those involved in competition during college years, may be quite different from active women.

Definitions

Terms must first be defined, for differences in definition alone may categorize a woman as eumenorrheic in some studies and as oligomenorrheic in others.

Common descriptors, agreed upon at this meeting, could help us compare studies with more meaning and confidence.

The term *regular* is most uniformly assigned to menstrual bleeding which occurs between 21 and 35 days, although some of the earlier research included several days on each end (Carlberg, Buckman, Peake, & Riedesel, 1983; Shangold, Freeman, Thysen, & Gatz, 1979). The parameters for irregularity, often referred to as *oligomenorrhea*, vary even more widely (see Table 1). Both the spacing between cycles and number of cycles per year that qualify a woman as being oligomenorrheic rather than amenorrheic differ. As is evident from Tables 2 and 3, the same women could be categorized in at least two different ways depending on the definition being used in that particular research study. Quite frequently oligo/amenorrheic women are combined in discussing data (Dale, Gerlach, & Wilhite, 1979; Wakat, Sweeney, & Rogol, 1982). Are they really the same? An underlying assumption that oligomenorrhea is an earlier phase of a continuum which leads to amenorrhea seems to be the most likely rationale for combining the two categories. The term *amenorrhea* also poses problems. Listed in Table 1 are differences in how researchers have defined this category.

A second set of definitions which confound the data concern body weight and body fat. The terms *underweight* and *underfat* are not easily comparable. Measurements of body fat have been shown to vary according to method. Studies in the literature have used at least four methods: hydrostatic underwater weighing, skinfold caliper measurements, estimation of body fat from the equation of Mellets and Cheek, and formulas using weight and height as criteria.

Exercise intensity must also be defined. In runners, is it the pace per mile or the number of miles run that is most likely to produce menstrual change? Does intense exercise for a trained woman have the same effect as for an untrained one? Does the stress induced by competition need to be measured, and if so, how?

Methodology

Methodology must also be considered in evaluating prevalence of menstrual change. The lowest prevalence has been reported in questionnaire studies. Questionnaire studies are open to criticism because they rely on a woman's recollection of her menstrual cycle. Women may report more regular cycles than would be documented with careful record keeping. In the past, questionnaire studies provided information that certain populations were less likely to exhibit menstrual change, but we have since learned that these figures must be substantiated by more complex data collection. Early questionnaire studies

Table 1

Classification of Menstrual Change

Investigator	Definition

A. Eumenorrhea—"Regular"

Gray	Recurrence of menstruation on a regular basis occurring at least nine times a year. (*Journal of Sport Science*, 1983)
Lutter	Women who regularly menstruate at least every 35 days; average 11 menstrual periods per year. (*The Physician and Sportsmedicine*, 1982)
Boyden	Consistent inter- and intracycle length without intracycle bleeding. (*Journal of Clinical Endocrinology and Metabolism*, 1982)
Bullen	Ovulatory character of the menstrual cycles confirmed by the findings of midluteal concentrations of plasma progesterone in the normal range. (*Sports Medicine—Sports Science*, 1983)
Bullen	Ovulatory functions and luteal phases of normal length (at least 9 days intervening between the LH surge and subsequent menses. (Conference on Menstrual Cycles and Physical Activity—Abstract, 1984)
Bonen	"Especially in athletic populations, the classification of menstrual cycles as 'normal' should be viewed with extreme skepticism in the absence of supporting endocrine data." (*The Physician and Sportsmedicine*, in press)

B. Oligomenorrhea—"Irregular"

Shangold	Inconsistent intervals of less than 23, more than 37 days, and less than 6 months (*American Journal of Obstetrics and Gynecology*, 1982)
Lutter	Continue to menstruate but at intervals greater than 35 days. (*The Physician and Sportsmedicine*, 1982)
Frisch	Intervals between menstruation of more than 38 days but less than 3 months. (*New England Journal of Medicine*, 1980)

Table 1 (Cont.)

Investigator	Definition
Gray	Irregular, infrequent (less than nine, but greater than four, per year) occurrence of menstruation after the establishment of regular menstrual cycles. (*Journal of Sport Science*, 1983)
Wakat	Reported a decreased frequency of menstrual cycles in the previous year with only one menstrual period within the last 3 months. (*Medicine and Science for Sport and Exercise*, 1982)
Boyden	Intercycle length increase or decrease; decrease in volume or number of days of blood loss. (*Journal of Clinical Endorinology and Metabolism*, 1982)

C. Amenorrhea

Investigator	Definition
Frisch	Lack of cycles for longer than 3 consecutive months. (*New England Journal of Medicine*, 1980)
Frisch	A 6-month interval between cycles. (*Journal of the American Medical Association*, 1981)
Carlberg	No menstrual periods during previous 3 months or four or fewer periods during the previous year. (*European Journal of Applied Physiology*, 1983)
Wakat	No period within last 6 months. (*Medicine and Science for Sport and Exercise*, 1982)
Gray	Decrease in occurrence of menstruation to three or fewer times per year after regular menstrual cycles had been established. (*Journal of Sport Science*, 1983)
Feicht	Three periods or less in 1 year. (*Lancet*, 1978)
Feicht Sanborn	Three or fewer menstrual periods a year. (*American Journal of Obstetrics and Gynecology*, 1982)
Shangold	No more than one bleeding episode during the prior 10 months. (*American Journal of Obstetrics and Gynecology*, 1982)

Table 2

Women Who Report Menstruating
at Irregular Intervals of Four Times Per Year

Classification	Investigator
Oligomenorrheic	Carlberg, Feicht, Lutter
Amenorrheic	Shangold, Gray
Questionable (dependent on interval)	Frisch, Wakat
Would not classify in absence of endocrine data	Bullen, Bonen, Boyden

and hormonal studies provided direction and hypotheses for our current work, but new studies must incorporate many measures to determine the dynamics of the changes taking place. Team approaches using experts from medical, physiological, nutritional, psychological, and statistical specialties have become a necessity. Deciding what methods and approaches are most likely to provide the needed data is another possible focus for this meeting.

Table 3

Women Reporting "Normal" Menses at 28-Day Intervals

Studies

"Regular"
   Questionnaire studies
   Endocrine studies which do not assess inter/intracycle length or luteal phase

"Questionable status"
   Until endocrine data available

Prevalence in Diverse Populations

Methodological problems so confound a discussion of prevalence in earlier studies that it is most appropriate to concentrate on several of the most recent studies which have documented change in the menstrual cycle. The several studies included here highlight the fact that prevalence will, to a large extent, be influenced by the population studied and the intensity of exercise.

Menstrual change, including anovulatory cycles and short luteal phase, is more likely to occur in young women who move from a moderately low level of physical fitness to a high level over a short period of time, as found in a study by Bullen, Beitins, Skrinar, & McArthur (1984). In this study, 25 subjects enrolled in a summer camp, with a mean age of 22.1 ± 0.5 years, gynecological age 9.5 ± 0.5 years, were studied over a 3-month period, which included a control month followed by 2 months of increasing exercise. Over a 2-month period, participants ran 20 mi in the first week, increasing the distance they were running to 50 mi in the fifth week. They continued to run at the 50-mi level in addition to engaging in other moderate activities such as swimming or biking for 3-1/2 hr/day. Morning weight and bedtime temperature were recorded, and a timed overnight urine specimen was collected to assess changes in the excretion of selected hormones (Bullen et al., 1982).

When 50 cycles were analyzed, only 2 women showed no menstrual change. In the first month, 4 women experienced anovulatory cycles; by the end of 2 months, 46% were anovulatory. Short luteal phase (22%), luteal insufficiency (24%), delayed menstruation (22%), hypomenorrhea (16%), and polymenorrhea (16%) were also documented (Bullen et al., 1984). Important nutritional and psychological data were also collected and are still being analyzed (B. Bullen, personal communication, February, 1984).

This study was described at some length to illustrate several important points:

1. Menstrual regularity as determined by endocrine status was confirmed before one could enter the study group.
2. Multiple factors could be controlled and monitored in the summer camp environment.
3. Under these circumstances, anovulatory cycles developed in 46% of the women: 22% exhibited short luteal phase, and 24% had measurable luteal insufficiency.
4. A 6-month follow-up was an important part of the study design (J. McArthur, personal communication, February, 1984); all subjects had returned to their pretraining menstrual characteristics 6 months later. A

critical question left unanswered, however, is what happened to exercise patterns in that 6-month period.

Prevalence patterns under laboratory or experimental conditions, however, should be generalized carefully to other populations. It is the rare woman who would increase her running and other exercise as quickly or as regularly as those in the Bullen et al. (1982) study.

Prior and colleagues report several studies that are useful in describing women who increased mileage over a longer time span. Using basal body temperature (BBT) and exercise training records for 14 women training for a marathon, Prior (1982) showed that one third of the 48 cycles recorded prior to the marathon were normal, one third showed shortened luteal phase, and one third were anovulatory. The women in this study had an average age of 36.0 ± 3.6 years (Prior, Pride, Vigna, & Yuen, 1983).

Another study by Prior (1982), where the conditions may be more applicable to a general population, involved four normally ovulating women who began a training program where they gradually increased distance from 5 to 12 km 5 days a week. One month of exercise was associated with significant shortening of the cycle length and a luteal phase shortened from 11.75 ± 0.5 days to 9.75 ± 2.2 days. Prior et al. (1982) also documented reversibility in two women who experienced anovulation and short luteal phase while in marathon training. Both women resumed regular ovulatory patterns when their running was greatly diminished or stopped. One of the women achieved pregnancy after 6 weeks and carried the baby uneventfully to term.

Another good example of change under less dramatic conditions is documented by Boyden et al. (1982). Women in this study increased their level of activity in a manner even more likely to be emulated by the average woman. Fourteen women, mean age 29.1 years, volunteered for a program designed to train them so that they could complete a marathon 14 to 15 months later. Boyden et al. used careful methods of determining ovulatory cycles, thereby assuring that change could be accurately documented. The 14 women increased their mileage from a mean of 15.1 ± 5.8 mi/week to 47.4 ± 5.7 mi/week at 30 weeks and 64.1 ± 7.0 mi/week at 50 weeks. Total body weight did not change, but there was significant loss of fat weight at 30 weeks and a significant increase in lean weight at 50 weeks.

At the end of the 50-week training period, 13 of the 14 participants had menstrual change, but none had amenorrhea. Menstrual changes included a decrease in volume or number of days of blood loss or both for 11 women. Intercycle length increased by 12 days and 16 days in 2 subjects and decreased by 5 and 11 days in 2 subjects; intermenstrual bleeding occurred in 2. Dysmenorrhea improved in 7 and worsened in 3 women. These studies have been presented to illustrate that prevalence will depend, in large part, not only on the population selected, but the exercise regime employed.

Prevalence and Persistence

Good documentation of increased prevalence of menstrual change is becoming available, particularly in certain populations under certain conditions. However, prevalence in several distinct populations must be further defined and an attempt must be made to predict prevalence for those girls and women who do not fit the patterns studied.

If a woman, particularly a young woman, increases her physical activity at a rapid rate, she is likely to experience menstrual change. The changes will probably be subtle at first and will be seen as shortened luteal phase. These changes will not be reported in a questionnaire study because most women will continue to bleed normally. These changes may, however, be detected by BBT or carefully described premenstrual symptoms. If new definitions of menstrual change that are based on luteal phase length are accepted, the prevalence in young women is probably higher than the 40 to 50% range reported in earlier studies. Evidence for new figures can be found in research reported by Bonen and Keizer (1984), who point out that one interpretation of Prior's data would suggest 66% of the participants showed shortened luteal phase although only 33% stopped bleeding.

The present level of knowledge suggests that older women who begin to train less rigorously will not experience the same dramatic changes as younger women, but further study is needed. If the phenomenon proves reliable, it implies that most women may avoid menstrual cycle change with less strenuous activity. This allows physicians to help individual women make important choices. For example, if a woman desires to become pregnant in the near future, she should be informed of the risk in moving from 15 mi/week of recreational running to 80 mi/week of marathon training. If, however, she is not desirous of pregnancy in the near future, there is little reason to avoid high-distance, high-intensity training and the possible 50% plus chance of decreased menses or shortened luteal phase. Researchers also need to further document prevalence of menstrual change in other sports so that women in their desired childbearing years might choose an activity less likely to contribute to menstrual change.

Much less is known about persistence of menstrual change than about prevalence. Most of the studies in the literature report that women experience some degree of reversibility when their exercise pattern decreases. This seems to be true even in the absence of significant changes in weight. Long-term follow-up studies that document the changes and their relationship to lifestyle and aging are needed. Recontacting some of the women in the early Dale and Wakat studies would provide valuable information on menstrual patterns over the ensuing years.

Very few women studied at Melpomene Institute have had long-term patterns of amenorrhea. After a year of concentrated effort to identify Twin Cities women who have had three or fewer periods in the previous 12 months, only

12 were located. While some may argue that women who do not experience such dramatic menstrual change must be considered, these are probably the women most at risk for other estrogen-deficiency problems. Persistence and possible long-term problems are the issues now demanding attention.

Amenorrhea:
Menstrual Dysfunction or Physiological Adaptation?

As studies have become more sophisticated, the definition of amenorrhea has been changing. Hormonal studies by Bonen and Keizer (1984), Prior (1982), Prior et al. (1982), and Prior et al. (1983) suggest that if BBT is considered, short luteal phases will be found in many women experiencing bleeding at regular intervals. These women believe they are having regular cycles and so may be recruited as controls or labeled as regular in studies which do not include BBT or hormonal analyses. Therefore, it may be decided that a luteal phase of at least 10 days is necessary before a woman is described as menstruating regularly (Bonen & Keizer, 1984). Another problem here is what Prior (1982) calls the dynamic dimension of menstruation: an individual may experience a variety of cycle types. When 11 women in her study submitted at least two cycles for review, 73% of the women had experienced both monophasic and biphasic cycles.

Defining regularity in terms of luteal phase may be appropriate for research design, as it has important implications in helping to understand the hormonal milieu. It presents major problems in reporting data which can be compared with the presumed "normal" nonexercising population because no one has collected data on the luteal phase of a large enough control group.

Researchers must also be concerned about the implications this use of terminology has for the way these menstrual changes are viewed. Is the discussion about menstrual dysfunction or physiological adaptation? The term *menstrual change* has purposely been used to avoid negative or positive connotations. Many of the published articles have clearly seen change as dysfunction and this is another issue that must be addressed.

Is the 28-day cycle of the Western woman really the ideal? Short (1978) and Ullyot (1981) have suggested that the number of cycle days common to a North American urban population differs greatly from that of African tribes where there seems to be a positive adaptation toward a minimum number of cycles throughout a woman's life span. Although most of the writing about amenorrhea continues to call it a problem or at least menstrual dysfunction, Short (1978) suggests that menstruation at 28-day cycles may be an "iatogenic disorder of civilized communities." Macvicar, Harlan, and Ouellet (1982) suggest that "there is an increasing tendency to view unique cycle variations from the perspective of health: that is a physiologically normal response to challenging stimuli."

Discussion

Those involved in research need to be aware of more complex health issues. The following questions must be answered:

1. What are the consequences of anovulatory cycles?
2. Will some women experience deleterious effects from long-term menstrual change? This may be a particularly important question for the woman who experiences long-term amenorrhea.
3. Are these menstrual changes reversible?
4. How can ovulatory cycles be stimulated?
5. When should an anovulatory woman who wishes to become pregnant in the future seek advice and possibly change her lifestyle?

Recommendations

Research that describes those women who might be most likely to experience menstrual change must be continued, keeping in mind that each woman probably has an individual threshold for the occurrence of oligo/amenorrhea. Do those individuals who have kept records and who can relate changes in training, diet, or stress to cycle changes control these aspects to prevent menstruation? Should they be encouraged to change patterns so that they menstruate a certain number of times per year?

Studies that clarify ideas and hypotheses such as those discussed in this paper are obviously necessary. Some of those already in progress have induced menstrual change with increased levels of training. Others are long-term studies which will document the natural course of amenorrhea to try to document reversibility. In all these new studies there has been increased sophistication of research design. This meeting can provide the opportunity to agree on basic definitions so that research findings can truly be compared and to agree that diverse populations need to be studied.

More frequent correspondence and discussion with each other are necessary so that efforts are not duplicated and ideas that may enhance a project in the early stages of development are quickly exchanged. Data must be presented carefully at conferences, in the scientific press, and in the popular press so that women are aware of possible problems connected with menstrual change and can find accurate information. Women who are unlikely to experience amenorrhea must not be unnecessarily alarmed any more than those experiencing long-term amenorrhea must not be ignored.

The prevalence question will remain a difficult one to answer definitively. Defining prevalence in subpopulations and determining its long-term importance is a challenge this meeting should help us achieve. Our direction for the future needs to focus on who is most susceptible and what long-term consequences are for that population.

References

Bonen, A., & Keizer, H.A. (1984). Athletic menstrual cycle irregularity: Endocrine response to exercise and training. *The Physician and Sportsmedicine*, **12**(8), 78-94.

Boyden, T.W., Pamenter, R.W., Grosso, D., Stanforth, P., Rotkis, T., & Wilmore, J.H. (1982). Prolactin responses, menstrual cycles and body composition of women runners. *Journal of Clinical Endocrinology and Metabolism*, **54**, 711-714.

Bullen, B.A., Beitins, I.Z., Carr, D.B., Skrinar, G.S., Orsulak, P.J., & McArthur, J.W. (1982). *Athletic stress and menstrual dysfunction. Sports medicine—sports science: Bridging the gap* (pp. 83-97). Lexington, MA: Collamore Press, D.C. Heath.

Bullen, B.A., Beitins, I.Z., Skrinar, G.S., & McArthur, J.W. (1984). Evolution of menstrual dysfunction with increased training severity. Conference on Menstrual Cycle and Physical Activity (ABST).

Carlberg, K.A., Buckman, M.T., Peake, G.T., & Riedesel, M.L. (1983). Menstrual function in athletes. *European Journal of Applied Physiology*, **51**, 211.

Dale, E., Gerlach, D.H., Wilhite, A.L. (1979). Menstrual dysfunction in distance runners. *Obstetrics and Gynecology*, **54**, 47-53.

Lutter, J.M., & Cushman, S. (1982). Menstrual patterns in female runners. *The Physician and Sportsmedicine*, **10**(9), 60-72.

Macvicar, M.G., Harlan, J.D., & Ouellet, M. (1982). What do we know about the effects of sports training on the menstrual cycle? *American Journal of Maternal Child Nursing*, **7**, 55-58.

Prior, J.C. (1982). Endocrine "conditioning" with endurance training: A preliminary review. *Canadian Journal of Applied Sport Science*, **7**(3), 148-157.

Prior, J.C., Pride, S., Vigna, Y., & Yuen, B.Ho. (1983). The marathon and reversible luteal phase shortening: A controlled prospective study. *Medicine and Science for Sports and Exercise*, **15**, 173 (ABST).

Prior, J.C., Yuen, B.Ho., Clement, P., Bowie, L., & Thomas, J. (1982, July). Infertility associated with marathon training. *Lancet,* pp. 269-270.

Shangold, M.M., Freeman, R., Thysen, B., & Gatz, M. (1979). The relationship between long-distance running, plasma progesterone, and luteal phase length. *Fertility and Sterility,* **31,** 130.

Short, R.V. (1978). Healthy infertility. *Upsala Journal of Medical Sciences Supplement,* **22,** 23-26.

Ullyot, J. (1981, December). Amenorrhea: A sensitive subject. *Women's Sports,* pp. 46-47.

Wakat, D.K., Sweeney, K.A., & Rogol, A.D. (1982). Reproductive system function in women cross-country runners. *Medicine and Science in Sports Exercise,* **14**(4), 263-269.

Reactions to Judy Mahle Lutter's Presentation

Reactor: Diane Wakat

The original study on the interaction of work (physical work) and the menstrual cycle was judged the Boylston Prize Essay in 1892 at Harvard University and was conducted by a physician named Mary Putnam Jacoby. Whereas she looked at the controversial question of the effect of the menstrual cycle on work capacity, we are looking at the influence of work on the menstrual cycle.

As in any emerging field of scientific endeavor, the initial reports tantalize, excite, and confuse us. It is now obvious that exercise of at least moderate intensity can, may, and does influence the function of the female reproductive system. But it is also obvious that drawing conclusions about prevalence and especially about the mechanism of exercise-induced menstrual cycle alteration (and I use the word *alteration* intentionally) is very difficult and perhaps hazardous at this point in time. This does not negate the value of previous research; that research has given us the forward direction that we need.

What information has the initial research provided to us and what is a good research design to precisely determine prevalence? To determine prevalence, we must define our terms according to endocrine criteria. We play games with words like *normal*, *nonnormal*, and *dysfunctional*. Everyone is saying "endocrine dysfunction." How do we know that? We need to

1. develop standard definitions (for "normal," etc.);
2. design our studies to elucidate the mechanism underlying effect of exercise on the reproductive system—not just *who* is affected but *why* and *how*;
3. carefully select subjects and controls that allow us to isolate the mechanism;
4. quantify exercise load so we can compare subjects and results;
5. monitor the many confounding variables; and
6. apply rigorous statistical and physiological research standards (for statistical significance and physiological relevance).

We have been very lax in defining what is normal. We no longer have that luxury. The definition of normal has to be standardized and it has to be measureable. I would suggest we use the term *eumenorrhea* synonomously with *normal* for research purposes. There have to be consistent criteria for a "menstrual cycle" (26 to 35 days), with appropriate division into follicular and luteal phases. We need to ensure that if subjects are normal, they have normal levels of hypothalamic, pituitary, and ovarian hormones, in proper sequence, in the right pattern and with the right amplitude. We need responsivity of target tissue to make sure the system works all the way down the line. We also need to make sure there is a functional brain, hypothalamic, pituitary, and gonadal axis. We must become more sophisticated in identifying the normal, unaffected female exerciser so that we can divide our groups for comparison. We have techniques to determine nonnormal patterns; we must utilize all of them.

Looking at the question of length of luteal phase, we may need to measure it by basal body temperature (which may not be 100% reliable) and level of hormones such as progesterone. We need to measure gonadotropin, specifically LH pulsatility by 24-hour measurement after Clomid induction, so that we can look at pituitary responsivity and hypothalamic function. We need to measure the pituitary response to gonadotropin releasing hormone. Is it responsive? How do we compare it to response of the normal person? We need to make sure there is ovarian responsivity. We may also need to determine by uterine histology that the person really has a functional axis.

That brings us to the question of how to select an appropriate control group. In many cases, the appropriate control is the person herself, because you know what the baseline is. Most of us have used eumenorrheic athletes in the same sport. Does that really tell us what we want to know about underlying mechanisms? Perhaps we should use endocrinologically dysfunctional females whom we know have certain lesions so that we can then compare and say, "Yes, this lesion is the same or is not the same." We need to look at symptoms, cycling and noncycling, indications of ovulation such as basal body temperature or hormone levels, follicular and luteal phase length, mean and integrated serum hormone levels, integrated and pulsatility measurements on these various hormones, and uterine histology. What this means is that a clinician has to be part of the team effort.

At present we have no standards to express exercise load. We talk about miles, hours, years, and "perceived exertion." We need to quantify exercise load by measuring intensity (METS or percent maxVO$_2$), duration, and frequency. We need some idea of the cumulative load in terms of years and the workout characteristics of the individual. The total number of subjects in our studies is going to have to increase so that we can statistically separate out the influence of different variables, and we need the help of people who know how to do metaanalysis.

We need to evaluate confounding variables like parity, use of oral contraceptives, and menstrual history. Menstrual history may indicate self-selection; girls with later menarche, may grow taller and become better volleyball players. Exercise intensity/load and training history are important. What may be a negative impact of exercise for one age group may be a positive impact in another age group. Level of competition (in terms of intensity of exercise and stress), body composition (percent fat as well as metabolic and nutritional considerations), and temperature are important. The susceptibility of individuals to competition and stress may vary, requiring the services of a sports psychologist.

We need to focus on the following three points: (a) basic physiology and endocrinology; (b) applied studies with practical considerations and advice for athletes; and (c) development of a susceptibility profile or a prediction equation for exercise effects. We need a multidisciplinary approach to studying eumenorrheic women engaged in quantified exercise regimens, so that we can construct a multidimensional picture of the influence of exercise intensity on women of varying ages with reproductive systems of varying susceptibility. Then we will be able to speak with authority about prevalence.

Discussion

Diane Wakat: Differences in reported prevalence are due to the fact that we have not used consistent definitions and that methodology has not been consistent. For example, there is a problem when using basal body temperature to assess the short luteal phase. Not all women are going to exhibit a thermogenic change in response to progesterone. Some women have a rise in basal body temperature a couple of days after ovulation has occurred. Thus, basal body temperature may not be an accurate method for assessing the short luteal phase.

Janet MacArthur: Not only do the definitions of cycle lengths and of disorders vary in the literature, but also the actual hormonal measurements vary from one woman to another. There is an exceedingly valuable paper reported in a recent symposium where a very large amount of information was amassed and showing how faithful a given woman is to her own control levels but how diverse the levels are from one woman to another.

Joan Ullyot: Doctors not really involved and who have not read the literature assume that any amenorrhea that occurs in a woman who exercises is athletic amenorrhea. Of course, there may be other factors—stress, weight loss, inadequate caloric intake, yes, even pregnancy. Thus, there may be clinical criteria for "true athletic amenorrhea" as opposed to amenorrhea in an athlete. It would be a great benefit if we could get some kind of pattern, some sort of fingerprint, of hormones which define athletic amenorrhea as opposed to other amenorrhea.

Diane Wakat: Right now we have the most data on two groups: college students and rats. We need to select other groups. Some women ask if they can use their amenorrhea as birth control. What you have to answer is "only if you run farther and faster."

4

Etiology of Athletic Amenorrhea

Charlotte Feicht Sanborn
University of Denver

Secondary amenorrhea is common among certain athletes. The fact that the highest frequencies have been noted primarily among runners and ballet dancers may provide a clue to the etiology of this disorder. These athletes characteristically have low body weight and low percent body fat (Frisch, Wyshak, & Vincent, 1980; Wilmore & Brown, 1974). The finding that secondary amenorrhea is a likely consequence of extreme thinness is rooted in sound clinical observations of disorders such as anorexia nervosa (Crisp & Stonehill, 1971). This has led to the most commonly held theory that athletic amenorrhea is caused by low body fat. The hypothesis is that when enough body fat is lost, the athlete falls below a critical percent fat and becomes amenorrheic. Because even the most casual observation shows that female distance runners and ballet dancers are quite slim, the fat hypothesis is intuitively attractive. Consequently, the majority of the current research in athletic amenorrhea has been directed toward testing the first logical piece of the puzzle. In the course of examining the role of body fat, however, confounding factors have emerged as additional potential causes of athletic amenorrhea. However, the fat hypothesis merits special attention not only for the amenorrheic athlete but also for its scientific value.

Fat Hypothesis

The fat hypothesis originated from the work of Frisch and associates at Harvard (Frisch, 1972, 1974; Frisch & McArthur, 1974; Frisch & Revelle, 1970, 1971a, 1971b; Frisch, Revelle, & Cook, 1973) who have advanced the hypothesis that a direct relationship exists between a critical amount of fat and the onset and maintenance of menstruation. The theory is based on the observation that menarche occurs at a critical weight (about 48 kg) rather than a specific age (Frisch, 1974; Frisch & Revelle, 1970, 1971b). This critical weight is extrapolated to represent a critical percentage of body fat through use of two separate height-weight nomograms (Frisch & McArthur, 1974; Frisch et al., 1973). In one nomogram, a minimal weight for height for onset of menstruation was extrapolated to about 17% body fat. The second nomogram indicated the critical weight for height necessary for maintenance of menstrual cycles was equivalent to about 22% body fat. Thus, age at menarche will occur at 17% body fat and secondary amenorrhea will develop when body fat is below 22%.

There is additional indirect evidence to support the fat hypothesis. First, compelling support comes from the clinical observation of amenorrhea in anorexia nervosa patients and in women with simple weight loss. McArthur, Johnson, Hourihan, and Alonso (1976) prescribed a diet which was adequate in protein, vitamins, and minerals to 9 amenorrheic patients. Upon regaining weight to an average of 96.6% of normal weight, amenorrhea reversed in all 9 patients. In patients with amenorrhea associated with simple weight loss, dietary intervention was also found to result in resumption of ovulatory cycles (Knuth, Hull, & Jacobs, 1977). A second line of evidence supporting the fat hypothesis is the fact that puberty in rats is reached at a specific body weight rather than a critical age (Kennedy & Mitra, 1963). Third, the steady decrease in age at menarche in the past century has been attributed to reaching the critical weight at an earlier age due to better nutrition than in the past (Tanner, 1962; Wyshak & Frisch, 1982). And fourth, aromatization of androgens to estrogen occurs in adipose tissue, providing an extragonadal source of estrogen (Yen & Jaffe, 1978).

Several criticisms (Reeves, 1979; Trussell, 1980) have been directed at the fat hypothesis. The major one (Mellits & Cheek, 1970) is that Frisch and co-workers estimated percent body fat from a height-weight equation rather than measuring it directly. Second, several investigators have not found regular menstrual cycles to resume once a critical weight was gained in anorectic women. Isaacs, Leslie, Gomez, and Bayliss (1980) did not find a restoration of menstruation following weight gain in 12 patients with anorexia nervosa. Initially, the patients were an average of 69.3% of ideal body weight. The amenorrhea persisted even after weight increased to an average of 91.2% of ideal weight. Similar results were reported by Katz, Boyar, Roffwarg, Hellman, and Weiner (1978), who studied 8 anorexia nervosa patients on ad lib diets.

They concluded that there was not a simple relationship between the restoration of menses and weight or fatness.

At least two possible explanations could be given for the disparity in the anorexia nervosa data. None of these studies measured percent body fat directly. Weight gain or loss was expressed as a percent of ideal body weight not in terms of fat weight as determined from hydrostatic weighing. Secondly, the explanation could be a purely nutritional one. Generally the diets of women with anorexia nervosa are unbalanced; it could be postulated that these women lack the necessary precursors for synthesis of hormones (Katz et al., 1978).

Female athletes, especially runners and ballet dancers, are excellent subjects for testing the fat hypothesis. Competitive distance runners have body fat levels as low as 5.9% (Wilmore & Brown, 1974). Preliminary findings in surveys of athletes tend to support the critical weight theory. Speroff and Redwine (1980) found that menstrual irregularities and amenorrhea were most common in runners who weighed less than 115 lbs and who lost more than 10 lbs after beginning training. Our group (Sanborn, Martin, & Wagner, 1982) found that in runners who had a higher prevalence of amenorrhea than in swimmers or cyclists there was a correlation between weight and amenorrhea. The lightest group of runners (less than 50 kg body weight) had higher levels of amenorrhea than women who weighed more than 50 kg (see Figure 1). Shangold and Levine (1982) also found amenorrheic runners to be

Figure 1

Runners were grouped into three body weight categories to examine the relationship of amenorrhea and weekly training mileage. The levels of athletic amenorrhea increased as the body weights of the runners decreased.

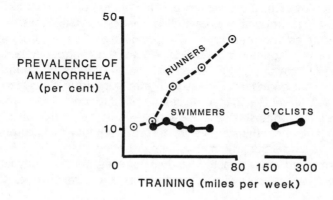

From "Is Athletic Amenorrhea Specific to Runners?" by C.F. Sanborn, B.J. Martin, and W.W. Wagner, 1982, *American Journal of Obstetrics and Gynecology*, **143**, p. 860. Reprinted with permission.

significantly lighter in body weight than regularly menstruating women (50 kg vs. 55 kg, respectively, $p < .05$). When Carlberg, Buckman, Peake, and Riedesel (1983b) surveyed 254 female athletes, low body weight was found to be the most important factor related to amenorrhea. Underweight athletes reported a higher frequency of amenorrhea than normal or overweight athletes.

Findings in ballet dancers with primary and secondary amenorrhea (Cohen, Kim, May, & Ertel, 1982; Frisch et al., 1980) further support the critical weight theory. These athletes were lower in body weight than the regularly menstruating ballet dancers (43.5 kg for primary amenorrhea, 44.9 kg for secondary amenorrhea, and 47.0 kg for regularly menstruating). Ballet dancers with secondary amenorrhea in the study by Cohen et al. also weighed less than regularly menstruating dancers. While average body weights were not provided, amenorrheic dancers had a significantly lower percent of ideal weight than dancers without menstrual irregularities (84.3% and 88.6%, respectively, $p < .05$).

Low body weight, however, is not always synonymous with low body fat. Many athletes may initially lose weight with training but weight then stabilizes; however, body fat can continue to decrease, resulting in an alteration of the lean mass to body fat ratio. Boyden et al. (1982) found that women training for a marathon had a decrease in percent fat without a change in body weight. A complex relationship exists between exercise and body composition. Thus, weight and height are not the most accurate predictors of body composition for athletes.

Recent studies have attempted to compare the percent body fat of amenorrheic and regularly menstruating athletes. Schwartz et al. (1981) compared amenorrheic runners (no menses for at least 4 months preceding the study) to three groups: (a) regularly menstruating runners who ran less than 30 mi/week, (b) regularly menstruating runners who ran more than 30 mi/week, and (c) nonrunning controls. Mean percent body fat and weight were significantly lower in the amenorrheic runners in comparison to the other groups ($p < .01$). Body fat was estimated from skinfold thicknesses and was 18.2% for the amenorrheic runners, approximately 23% for both groups of regularly menstruating runners and 27.4% for the controls. Baker, Mathur, Kirk, and Williamson (1981) studied 23 women runners and found that the average percent body fats as measured from skinfold thicknesses were not statistically different (14.1% for the amenorrheic runners, 17.7% for regularly menstruating runners). Wakat, Sweeney, and Rogol (1982) also found no significant differences in mean weight or sum of skinfold thicknesses between amenorrheic and regularly menstruating runners. Using the hydrostatic weighing method with estimated residual volumes, percent body fat was not different between dancers with and without menstrual irregularities (Calabrese et al., 1983).

Opposite results were found by Carlberg, Buckman, Peake, and Riedesel (1983a) in a group of 42 female athletes. These athletes were selected from college varsity sports (track and field, swimming and diving, tennis, and volleyball), high school varsity track and field, and a general population of distance runners. Percent body fat was measured by the hydrostatic weighing technique using a helium dilution method to calculate residual volume. The amenorrheic athletes (no menses in the previous 3 months or less than four periods in the previous year) had a significantly lower percent body fat (13.1%) than the regularly menstruating group (16.3%, $p < .05$). However, a considerable amount of overlap between the two groups was found. Amenorrheic athletes had a range of body fat from 7 to 18% and the regularly menstruating athletes had an even greater scatter from 8 to 27%. Because of the large overlap, the authors concluded that there is no critical level of body fat as hypothesized for athletic amenorrhea. Instead, they proposed an individual set-point for each athlete as a possible explanation.

These studies of body fat and athletic amenorrhea have produced conflicting results. There were important differences in methods. Three studies used skinfold thickness measurements and the other two used hydrostatic weighing. Predictions of body density from anthropometric variables such as skinfold measurements are population-specific and can result in large prediction error (Jackson & Pollock, 1977). Although underwater weighing or hydrostatic weighing is one of the most accurate methods to date for measuring body density, accurate measurement of the residual lung volume is crucial for computing accurate body densities. Predicted values for residual volumes have a greater standard error than actual measured volumes ($\pm$ 500 ml, $\pm$ 100 ml, respectively), according to Wilmore (1969). For a 55 kg woman, the estimation of body fat could have an error of $\pm$ 5% using a predicted residual volume.

Understanding the role of body fat and body weight in athletic amenorrhea is further complicated by the existence of confounding variables such as late menarche, intense training prior to menarche, prior menstrual irregularities, immature reproductive axis, intense training, and psychological stress. Because these factors continually surface, each has been implicated with the onset of amenorrhea in athletes.

Late Menarche

A later age of menarche has been reported for athletes than for nonathletes (Malina, Harper, Avent, & Campbell, 1973). The mean age of menarche was 13.6 years for 66 college track and field athletes and 12.2 years for 30 nonathletes, a significant difference. Malina, Spirduso, Tate, and Baylor (1978) reported that Olympic volleyball athletes had a significantly later age at menarche (14.2 years) compared to high school and college athletes (13.0 years) and controls (12.3 years). Amenorrheic ballet dancers also have delayed menarche. Menarche usually occurred at age 14 years for the amenorrheic ballet dancers (Calabrese, 1983; Frisch et al., 1980); an even later age of 15 years was reported by Warren (1980).

Among amenorrheic runners the findings have been diverse. Feicht, Johnson, Martin, Sparks, and Wagner (1978) reported a significantly delayed menarche in amenorrheic middle-distance runners (14.1 yrs) versus the regularly menstruating group (13.3 yrs). A similar later age of menarche was reported by Wakat, Sweeney, and Rogol (1982) in their amenorrheic runners: 14.3 years compared to 12.9 years for the regularly menstruating runners. Baker et al. (1981) found that the age of menarche was significantly higher in amenorrheic runners (13.8 years) than in regularly menstruating runners (12.2 years). On the other hand, two studies on runners have found the age at menarche to be similar between the two groups. Schwartz et al. (1981) reported a mean menarcheal age of 12.8 years for all the athletes and Shangold and Levine (1982) found menarche to occur at age 12.2 years for the amenorrheic runners and 12.7 years for the regularly menstruating runners. The cause of late menarche in some athletes is not known.

Malina et al. (1978) raised an interesting question about late menarche. Does athletic training delay menarche, or do late maturers choose to be in certain sports? Frisch et al. (1981) examined the relationship between age at menarche and age at initiation of training. They reported that for each year of training before puberty, menarche was delayed 5 months. Malina (1982) urged caution in interpreting these results because the conclusions were based on small numbers and indicated a correlation, not a cause-and-effect relationship. Vandenbrouch, vanLaar, and Valkenburg (1982) not only found that intense sports activity alone could delay menarche but that a synergistic effect occurred between sports participation and thinness in delaying menarche. How late menarche might be linked to athletic amenorrhea is not known. Perhaps a late age of menarche implies an immature reproductive endocrine axis which would be prone toward menstrual changes.

Prior Menstrual Irregularities

Secondary amenorrhea has been reported to be more common in athletes who had a history of prior menstrual irregularities. Shangold and Levine (1982) stated that the single best predictor of amenorrhea in their sample of runners was prior menstrual irregularities. Schwartz et al. (1981) found that over 50% of their amenorrheic runners had past menstrual cycle irregularities.

Immature Reproductive Endocrine Axis

Dale, Gerlach, and Wilhite (1979) were the first to suggest that athletic amenorrhea may be a result of an immature reproductive endocrine axis. Their suggestion was based on the finding that prior pregnancy appeared to be related to regularity. Fifty percent of the runners who had never borne children (nulliparous) had menstrual irregularities while only 20% of the parous runners developed irregularities. The maturity of the hypothalamic-pituitary-ovarian system has also been related to age of the athlete. Baker et al. (1981) found that amenorrhea occurred more often in runners who were younger than 30 years of age (66.6%) than in those 30 years of age or greater (9.0%). These findings suggest that younger, nulliparous runners may be more susceptible to athletic amenorrhea because of an immature hypothalamic-pituitary-ovarian axis. These data support the observations of Erdelyi (1962) and Speroff and Redwine (1980) that younger women are more susceptible to menstrual dysfunction.

Intense Training

The frequency of amenorrhea has been positively correlated with the number of miles run per week. The prevalence steadily increased from 6% in those running the least to 43% in those running more than 60 miles per week (Feicht et al., 1978). In a later study, Sanborn, Martin, and Wagner (1982) surveyed runners, cyclists, and swimmers to determine the prevalence of amenorrhea in these endurance sports. Again weekly training mileage was correlated with amenorrhea among the runners; however, no such relationship existed for the swimmers and cyclists (see Figure 2). An association between training and frequency of menstrual dysfunction in distance runners was substantiated by Dale et al. (1979). In this study, none of the controls (n = 54) experienced amenorrhea (0-5 periods per year) while 24% of the female distance runners did. Final support for a correlation was reported by Frisch et al. (1981) who found that training was associated with an increase in the prevalence of amenorrhea in swimmers (n = 21) and runners (n = 17).

In contrast, Wakat et al. (1982) found no greater prevalence of amenorrhea in the high-mileage groups than in any other group of cross-country runners. Disagreement between these studies could be a result of how the groups of athletes were divided. In the Feicht et al. (1978) and Sanborn et al. (1982) studies, each point on the graph (see Figures 1 and 2) represented an equal number of respondents, not a set range of miles run per week. In the Wakat et al. study, each point on the graph was selected based on an interval of 15 mi run per week. The number of athletes represented by each point is not known. Speroff and Redwine (1980) also found no correlation between weekly mileage running and amenorrhea. However, few of their women ran more than 20 mi/week. Finally, the effect of endurance training on the menstrual cycle was studied in 19 regularly menstruating women (Boyden et al., 1982). After approximately 13.5 months of training, the subjects were averaging 63.4 mi of running per week. Menstrual changes occurred in all

Figure 2

The prevalence of amenorrhea increases linearly as training mileage increases in runners (*p* < .001). Swimmers and cyclists have a 12% prevalence regardless of training mileage.

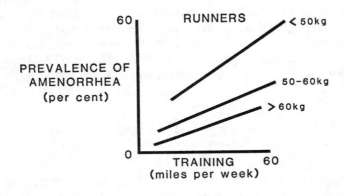

From "Is Athletic Amenorrhea Specific to Runners?" by C.F. Sanborn, B.J. Martin, and W.W. Wagner, 1982, *American Journal of Obstetrics and Gynecology*, **143**, p. 860. Reprinted with permission.

but one subject. The major change reported was a decrease in amount of menstrual flow and/or a decrease in number of days of menstruation. None of the subjects developed amenorrhea.

All of these studies have examined only duration of training in miles trained per week or the number of days, weeks, and months of training. None have examined the intensity of training, that is, training pace. In general, there seems to be an association between athletic amenorrhea and training mileage, especially in runners. However, until all parameters of training are examined, the role of athletics in amenorrhea will remain a mystery.

Psychological Stress

An alternative explanation for athletic amenorrhea could be stress stemming from intense training and competition. Support for this theory is shown in the following data. Amenorrheic middle-distance runners have subjectively rated the months they trained per year more intense than did the regularly menstruating group (Feicht et al., 1978). This finding was further substantiated by the work of Schwartz et al. (1981). Their group of amenorrheic athletes also subjectively evaluated their running to be associated with stress more than the regularly menstruating group. Four psychological tests were also administered to the athletes to assess depression, anxiety, compulsive behavior, hypochondriac tendencies, and overall stress. No significant differences were found between the groups for any of the objective tests. The reason provided by the authors for not finding similar results with the objective tests as in the subjective ratings was that the objective tests were not as sensitive for picking up subtle psychological differences.

In a study by Galle, Freeman, Galle, Huggins, & Sondheimer (1983), the Hopkins Symptom Checklist was used to evaluate psychological stress. Amenorrheic runners had higher scores for obsessive-compulsive behavior than regularly menstruating runners although all the scores were within the normal range. Opposite results have also been reported. Carlberg et al. (1983) interviewed amenorrheic athletes and athletes with irregular menstruation to determine factors that were associated with the menstrual dysfunction. Emotional stress was found to play a relatively minor role in the development of exercise-associated menstrual irregularities. Similar results were found by Gray and Dale (1983) among runners. Using the Schedule of Recent Experiences questionnaire, they found that stress was not correlated with the number of menstrual cycles per year.

Diet

There is accumulating evidence that nutritional status and diet affect the reproductive system. While the mechanisms for the dysfunction is unknown, poor dietary habits are often cited as the explanation for amenorrhea in anorexia nervosa. Protein deficiency, severe reduction of carbohydrate intake (Crisp & Stonehill, 1971), or red meat and fish intake (Knuth, Hull, & Jacobs, 1977), and elevated levels of carotene (Kemmann, Pasquale, & Skaf, 1983) have been implicated in the onset of secondary amenorrhea. Diet has also been linked to the production and excretion of estrogen hormones in women. Goldin et al. (1982) found that vegetarian women excreted more estrogens, resulting in a lower plasma concentration of estrogen than in omnivores. In this study the vegetarians consumed less total fat and more dietary fiber than the nonvegetarians.

The role of diet in athletic amenorrhea is unknown. Schwartz et al. (1981) evaluated 7-day, self-reported diets of regularly menstruating and amenorrheic runners. Even though the amenorrheic runners had a higher caloric intake, they had a lower protein intake than the cyclic runners. The data are only preliminary; further investigation is needed to clarify the association between diet and athletic amenorrhea.

Summary

The prevalence of secondary amenorrhea in athletes has encouraged investigation of the etiology of athletic amenorrhea. Because distance runners and ballet dancers have the highest frequencies of athletic amenorrhea and are characteristically low in body weight and body fat, a "fat hypothesis" has evolved. Two major lines of evidence have been used to support this hypothesis: (a) menarche occurs at a critical weight, and (b) some patients with anorexia nervosa begin menstruating after regaining weight. Data on body weights of amenorrheic athletes have tended to support the critical weight theory. Amenorrheic athletes weigh less than those with regular menstrual cycles. Findings on percent body fat, however, are conflicting. There are at least two reasons for this disagreement. First, percent body fat has been calculated using two different methods: skinfold thicknesses and hydrostatic weighing. In the latter measurement, additional error could result from using predicted versus actual measured residual volume. Second, confounding factors have existed in every study: late menarche, intense training prior to menarche, prior menstrual irregularities, intense training, immature reproductive axis, and psychological stress. These variables alone or in various combinations have been implicated in the development of athletic amenorrhea. At this time there is no clearcut explanation for the occurrence of athletic amenorrhea; the field is in ferment and represents a superb opportunity for further research.

References

Baker, E.R., Mathur, R.S., Kirk, R.F., & Williamson, H.O. (1981). Female runners and secondary amenorrhea: Correlation with age, parity, mileage, and plasma hormonal and sex-hormone-binding globulin concentrations. *Fertility and Sterility*, **36**, 183-187.

Boyden, T.W., Parmenter, R.W., Grosso, D., Stanforth, P., Rotkis, T., & Wilmore, J.H. (1982). Prolactin responses, menstrual cycles, and body composition of women runners. *Journal of Clinical Endocrinology and Metabolism*, **54**, 711-714.

Calabrese, L.H., Kirkendall, D.T., Floyd, M., Rapoport, S., Williams, G.W., Weiker, G.G., & Bergfeld, J.A. (1983). Menstrual abnormalities, nutritional patterns and body composition in female classical ballet dancers. *The Physician and Sportsmedicine*, **11**, 86-98.

Carlberg, K.A., Buckman, M.T., Peake, G.T., & Riedesel, M.L. (1983a). Body composition of oligo/amenorrheic athletes. *Medicine and Science in Sports and Exercise*, **15**, 215-217.

Carlberg, K.A., Buckman, M.T., Peake, G.T., & Riedesel, M.L. (1983b). A survey of menstrual function in athletes. *European Journal of Applied Physiology*, **51**, 211-222.

Cohen, J.L., Kim, C.S., May, P.B., & Ertel, N.H. (1982). Exercise, body weight, and amenorrhea in professional ballet dancers. *The Physician and Sportsmedicine*, **10**, 92-101.

Crisp, A.H., & Stonehill, C. (1971). Relation between aspects of nutritional disturbance and menstrual activity in primary anorexia nervosa. *The British Medical Journal*, **3**, 149-151.

Dale, E., Gerlach, D.H., & Wilhite, A.L. (1979). Menstrual dysfunction in distance runners. *Obstetrics and Gynecology*, **54**, 47-53.

Erdelyi, G.J. (1962). Gynecological survey of female athletes. *The Journal of Sports Medicine and Physical Fitness*, **2**, 174-179.

Feicht, C.B., Johnson, T.S., Martin, B.J., Sparks, K.E., & Wagner, W.W. (1978). Secondary amenorrhea in athletes. *Lancet*, **2**, 1145-1146.

Frisch, R.E. (1972). Weight at menarche: Similarity for well-nourished and undernourished girls at differing ages, and evidence for historical constancy. *Pediatrics*, **50**, 445-450.

Frisch, R.E. (1974). A method of prediction of age of menarche from height and weight at ages 9 through 13 years. *Pediatrics*, **53**, 384-390.

Frisch, R.E., Gotz-Welbergen, A.V., McArthur, J.W., Albright, T., Witschi, J., Bullen, B., Birnholz, J., Reed, R.B., & Hermann, H. (1981). Delayed menarche and amenorrhea of college athletes in relation to age of onset of training. *Journal of the American Medical Association*, **246**, 1559-1563.

Frisch, R.E., & McArthur, J.W. (1974). Menstrual cycles: Fatness as a determinant of minimum weight for height necessary for their maintenance or onset. *Science*, **185**, 949-951.

Frisch, R.E., & Revelle, R. (1970). Height and weight at menarche and a hypothesis of critical body weights and adolescent events. *Science*, **169**, 397-399.

Frisch, R.E., & Revelle, R. (1971a). The height and weight of girls and boys at the time of initiation of the adolescent growth spurt in height and weight and the relationship to menarche. *Human Biology*, **43**, 140-159.

Frisch, R.E., & Revelle, R. (1971b). Height and weight at menarche and a hypothesis of menarche. *Archives of Disease in Childhood, 46,* 695-701.

Frisch, R.E., Revelle, R., & Cook, S. (1973). Components of weight at menarche and the initiation of the adolescent growth spurt in girls: Estimated total water, lean body weight and fat. *Human Biology, 45,* 469-483.

Frisch, R.E., Wyshak, G., & Vincent, L. (1980). Delayed menarche and amenorrhea in ballet dancers. *New England Journal of Medicine, 303,* 17-19.

Galle, P.C., Freeman, E.W., Galle, M.G., Huggins, G.R., & Sondheimer, J.J. (1983). Physiologic and psychologic profiles in a survey of women runners. *Fertility and Sterility, 39*(5), 633-639.

Goldin, B.R., Adlercreutz, H., Gorbach, S.I., Warram, J.H., Dwyer, J.T., Swenson, L., & Woods, M.N. (1982). Estrogen excretion patterns and plasma levels in vegetarian and omnivorous women. *New England Journal of Medicine, 307,* 1542-1547.

Gray, D.P., & Dale, E. (1983). Variables associated with secondary amenorrhea in women runners. *Journal of Sports Sciences, 1,* 55-67.

Isaacs, A.J., Leslie, R.D., Gomez, J., & Bayliss, R. (1980). The effect of weight gain on gonadotropins and prolactin in anorexia nervosa. *Acta Endocrinologica, 94,* 145-150.

Jackson, A.S., & Pollock, M.L. (1977). Prediction accuracy of body density, lean body weight, and total body volume equations. *Medicine and Science in Sports, 9,* 197-201.

Katz, J.L., Boyar, R., Roffwarg, H., Hellman, L., & Weiner, H. (1978). Weight and circadian luteinizing hormone secretory pattern in anorexia nervosa. *Psychosomatic Medicine, 40,* 549-567.

Kennedy, G.G., & Mitra, J. (1963). Body weight and food intake as initiating factors for puberty in the rat. *Journal of Physiology (London), 166,* 408-418.

Kemman, E., Pasquale, S.A., & Skaf, R. (1983). Amenorrhea associated with carotenemia. *Journal of the American Medical Association, 249,* 926-929.

Knuth, U.A., Hull, M.G., & Jacobs, H.S. (1977). Amenorrhea and loss of weight. *British Journal of Obstetrics and Gynecology, 84,* 801-807.

Malina, R.M., Harper, A.B., Avent, H.H., & Campbell, D.E. (1973). Age at menarche in athletes and non-athletes. *Medicine and Science in Sports, 5,* 11-13.

Malina, R.M., Spirduso, W.W., Tate, C., & Baylor, A.M. (1978). Age at menarche and selected menstrual characteristics in athletes at different competitive levels and in different sports. *Medicine and Science in Sports, 10,* 218-222.

Malina, R.M. (1982). Delayed age of menarche of athletes. *Journal of American Medical Association,* **247,** 3312.

McArthur, J.W., Johnson, L., Hourihan, J., & Alonso, C. (1976). Endocrine studies during the refeeding of young women with nutritional amenorrhea and infertility. *Mayo Clinic Proceedings,* **51,** 607-616.

McArthur, J.W., Bullen, B.A., Beitins, I.Z., Pagano, M., Badger, M., & Klibanski, A. (1980). Hypothalamic amenorrhea in runners of normal body composition. *Endocrine Research Communications,* **7,** 89-91.

Mellits, E.B., & Cheek, D.B. (1970). The assessment of body water and fatness from infancy to adulthood. *Monographs of the Society for Research in Child Development,* **35**(7), 12-26.

Reeves, J. (1979). Estimating fatness. *Science,* **204,** 881.

Sanborn, C.F., Martin, B.J., & Wagner, W.W. (1982). Is athletic amenorrhea specific to runners? *American Journal of Obstetrics and Gynecology,* **143,** 859-861.

Schwartz, B., Cumming, D.C., Riordan, E., Selye, M., Yen, S.S., & Rebar, R.W. (1981). Exercise-associated amenorrhea: A distinct entity? *American Journal of Obstetrics and Gynecology,* **141,** 662-670.

Shangold, M.M., & Levine, H.S. (1982). The effect of marathon training upon menstrual function. *American Journal of Obstetrics and Gynecology,* **143,** 862-869.

Speroff, L., & Redwine, D.B. (1980). Exercise and menstrual function. *The Physician and Sportsmedicine,* **8,** 42-52.

Tanner, J.M. (1962). *Growth at adolescence* (2nd ed.). Oxford: Blackwell Scientific Publications.

Trussell, J. (1980). Statistical flaws in evidence for the Frisch hypothesis that fatness triggers menarche. *Human Biology,* **52,** 711-720.

Vandenbroucke, J.P., vanLaar, A., & Valkenburg, H.A. (1982). Synergy between thinness and intensive sports activity in delaying menarche. *British Medical Journal,* **284,** 1907-1908.

Wakat, D.K., Sweeney, K.A., & Rogol, A.D. (1982). Reproductive system function in women cross-country runners. *Medicine and Science in Sports and Exercise,* **14,** 263-269.

Warren, M.P. (1980). The effects of exercise on pubertal progression and reproductive function in girls. *Journal of Clinical Endocrinology and Metabolism,* **51,** 1150-1156.

Wentz, A. (1980). Body weight and amenorrhea. *Obstetrics and Gynecology,* **56,** 482-487.

Wilmore, J. (1969). The use of actual, predicted and constant residual volumes in the assessment of body composition by underwater weighing. *Medicine and Science in Sports,* **1,** 87-90.

Wilmore, J., & Brown, C. (1974). Physiological profiles of women distance runners. *Medicine and Science in Sports,* **6,** 178-181.

Wyshak, G., & Frisch, R.E. (1982). Evidence for a secular trend in age of menarche. *The New England Journal of Medicine,* **306,** 1033-1035.

Yen, S.C., & Jaffe, R.B. (1978). *Reproductive endocrinology.* Philadelphia: W.B. Saunders Co.

Reactions to
Charlotte Feicht Sanborn's Presentation

Reactor: Joel Stager

The evidence for the association between fatness and athletic amenorrhea is far from convincing. The effect of routine physical training upon body fatness is well known. Exercise alters the lean to fat ratio in favor of lean body mass increase and body fat mass decrease. Thus, any changes that occur as a result of physical training will appear to correlate with changes in fatness. The relationship between performance and physical activities wherein the body must be lifted or moved against gravitational force has been characterized numerous times. When considering body composition as a potential variable affecting menstrual periods, it might be wiser to consider athletic populations where body fat has little to do with athletic performance. Those studies using the more accepted (not necessarily state of the art), reliable techniques such as densitometry and skinfolds do not support the existence of a critical fatness variable in the etiology of athletic amenorrhea. Longitudinal studies where athletes have been followed for some period of time, either for hormone profiles or changes in body composition, tend to refute the fatness hypothesis. The reversibility of changes in menstrual function appear to occur prior to any detectable changes in composition. The rate at which menstrual cycles return following the cessation of training tends to discount the importance of body composition. This suggests that activity during critical phases of the cycle may be significant. This is not to say, however, that body composition is not important in reproductive function or development. That there is a variable, individually specific set point for body composition is possible, but currently seems unlikely.

Another issue deals with the use of measured versus estimated residual volumes when predicting body density. Clinically, or when working with a single individual, lung volumes are often estimated with the aid of a nomogram or prediction equation. Estimation of residual volume incurs an error of 5% body fat. But this error can be positive or negative; thus a larger population better estimates the mean. It is doubtful that predicting residual volume incurs large errors in the estimate of body composition when working with large populations.

That late menarche and athletic amenorrhea are related appears clear. That there is a causal relationship, however, remains to be shown. Correlation in this case does not imply causation. "Later" menarche is a more acceptable term. Again, we must be aware that athletic populations are prone to selection. That later menarche in athletes is caused by prepubertal athletic participation is highly suspect. The older the woman is at menarche, the more likely it is that training will begin prior to menarche and vice versa.

My final comment concerns the concept of training mileage and differences in the incidence of amenorrhea among different athletic populations. The definition of amenorrhea might change with different types of studies. In a comparison made at our lab, swimmers and runners were equally as likely to exhibit changes in menstrual periods, if we can consider oligomenorrhea of less than nine menses per year as the only criteria. However, if we restrict our definition of amenorrhea to fewer than three menses per year, the runners do indeed show a greater incidence of amenorrhea. However, in my opinion, this is due to the seasonal nature of the sport rather than a difference between runners and swimmers or differences in the effects of their exercise regimes. In summary, the existence of the relationship between athletic amenorrhea and body composition seems tenuous.

Measurement of residual volume is preferable for population studies, but it is unlikely that large errors are incurred by using a predicted equation. Let us not disregard these studies. "Later" menarche (rather than the term "delayed" menarche) appears to be associated with menstrual irregularity in athletes. That this is a causal relationship is doubtful. A definition is needed for oligomenorrhea and amenorrhea for further comparisons in future research. The concept of average weekly training mileage needs further thought—what may be a useful index in one sport may be less than a viable concept in another.

Discussion

Leonard Calabrese: Although my own study using densitometry with dancers failed to show any statistical difference between the regularly menstruating females and the nonregularly menstruating females, this does not discredit percent body fat as an important etiological agent in the development of menstrual problems. Failure to achieve statistical significance just means that these groups cannot be segregated by that one variable. The point made earlier in the review of endocrine function was that this is a marvelous common-sense type of adaptation that women appear to have. I think we should think more in terms of cofactors as opposed to single causes of this dysfunction. I think that emotional stress is an incredibly important factor in the development of these problems. It is the most poorly understood factor and the one least capable of quantification. A study of music students (by Gardner and Garfinkel) who are known to be under emotional stress resulted in no correlation between stress and abnormal periods compared to controls. Anderson studied women attending West Point (a very stressful situation) to examine effects of mixing emotional stress with exercise. So, perhaps there are combinations of factors. We should keep looking at other groups besides runners and dancers. People who have only one risk factor may be able to be segregated out.

Alan Rogel: Do equations for calculating body density from underwater weighing differ for a 67-year-old osteoporotic woman and a 19-year-old mesomorphic swimmer? And if they don't differ, could part of the reason be variability?

Charlotte Sanborn: The equations should be different because of differences in bone density. That could account for a lot of the differences we find between studies.

Karen Carlberg: I am going to disagree with Joel Stager. We should consider not just percent body fat but what that means in absolute terms of fat tissue and lean tissue. As Dr. Sanborn pointed out, in my study there was not a big difference in percent body fat between amenorrheic and menstruating athletes. But when I compared absolute amount of fat tissue and absolute amount of lean tissue, there was a much larger and highly significant difference. If we want to hypothesize that the relationship between menstrual characteristics and body composition is related to peripheral steroid metabolism, the absolute amounts of the tissue are a lot more important than just the percentage.

Joel Stager: Dr. Frisch's original hypothesis was somewhat similar to what you are saying in that it wasn't necessarily the percent of body fat that was important but the weight of fat which represented so many calories or stores of energy. And this stored energy was what was necessary as far as continuing or maintaining a pregnancy without endangering the health of the mother.

Arend Bonen: Peripheral steroid conversion does occur in muscle and we tend to forget about that. Thinking very simplistically about weight changes or body fat changes implies that there is somewhat of a negative caloric balance in the individual. When you get a negative caloric balance, there are tremendous metabolic changes occurring. It seems to me that some of these metabolic changes in terms of hormones, substrates, or what have you, somehow get back to the pituitary and hypothalamus. It may be that clinically the loss of body fat is a useful index. But can we say this is the cause of amenorrhea?

Blake Surina: The high school women gymnasts in our study were quite a bit lower in residual volume than the average sedentary person. Some people are more comfortable underwater and they have better ventilatory muscles and can blow out more air. Wilmore's 1983 review suggests taking x-rays and estimating bone density through radiography.

Chris Cann: We are going to cover some methodological issues later. We have been using CT scans to measure body fat and residual volume. We found that in older or normal control populations, the ratio of subcutaneous to intra-abdominal fat (something people really haven't looked at) is around 1.4 in females and it covers a wide range from very obese down to the athletes. When a change in subcutaneous fat is observed, skinfold measurements may be better than hydrostatic weighing because they appear to correlate better with the actual changes in body fat.

5

Hormonal Mechanisms of Reproductive Function and Hypothalamic Adaptation to Endurance Training

Jerilynn C. Prior
University of British Columbia

The process of reproduction involves the coordinated and integrated action of more than 12 hormones in the brain, the pituitary, and the ovary. Although reproduction is crucial for the species, continuous potential fertility is not essential for the individual. Therefore, when an individual's homeostasis is under challenge, temporary suppression of cyclic menstrual function may occur. The complex process of reproduction will be examined to set the stage for understanding how the menstrual cycle may change with physical activity.

Hypothalamic Neuroendocrine Regulation

Between menstrual bleeding at the beginning of one cycle and flow at the next, an incredible hormonal explosion occurs. The events at the midcycle

This work would not have been possible without the early cooperation of Drs. Basil Ho Yuen and Laura Jensen, the time and enthusiasm of Jo Thomas, and the perspicacity of Yvette Vigna. Thanks to Hazel Netterfield for transforming ideas into written words.

are largely unperceived by the woman, and poorly understood by neuroendocrinologists and gynecologists. Debate has raged in the last few years concerning primary responsibility for the timing and control of this great hormonal surge. Although hormones of the hypothalamus are essential, it appears from Knobil's (1980) work that the ovary plays an important regulatory role. He has shown that the dominant follicle of the ovary determines the timing and magnitude of the surge of luteinizing hormone (LH) and follicle stimulating hormone (FSH) at midcycle.

We must begin somewhere to describe the complex monthly chain of reproductive events. The logical place to start is in the center of the head, in a richly vascular area which has nerve connections to the major areas of the brain. The hypothalamus is strategically located in a nerve and hormonal network with links to the limbic system where emotions are interpreted. This small area above the pituitary, lying at the base of the brain, is responsible for temperature regulation, the integrated response to fasting and feeding, respiration, and pituitary hormonal regulation. Neuroendocrine control of reproduction has recently been reviewed (Yen, 1982) (see Figure 1). The major hypothalamic hormone of reproduction is gonadotropin-releasing hormone (GnRH). This ten-amino acid peptide, originally isolated in 1971 by Schally (1973) was synthesized shortly thereafter for clinical use. GnRH, produced in the arcuate nucleus of the hypothalamus, is secreted into the pituitary portal system and bathes the gonadotropin-producing cells (which make LH and FSH) of the pituitary.

Awakening of quiescent GnRH secretion determines the time of maturation to adulthood. During adult life in both men and women, GnRH exhibits a steady baseline secretion with approximate hourly bursts (circhoral rhythm) (Elkind-Hirsch, Ravinkar, Shift, Tulchinsky, & Ryan, 1982; Knobil, 1980). Prior to puberty, however, GnRH is present but is secreted in low nonpulsatile amounts. In the early stages of puberty, LH (and presumably GnRH) pulses begin to occur during sleep (Boyer, 1978). As puberty progresses, the timing of GnRH secretion matures to the adult circhoral pattern.

Further evidence for the role of GnRH in events initiating puberty can be shown by studies in young women with anorexia nervosa. These women had an absence of LH pulsation, but returned, following hourly GnRH injections, to a pubertal pattern of bursts of LH during sleep (Marshall & Kelch, 1979). Recent work documented that women with hypothalamic amenorrhea and infertility developed normal pulsatile patterns of LH and FSH and ovulatory menses in response to therapeutic GnRH administered in hourly pulses (Crowley & McArthur, 1980).

The hypothalamic message about reproduction is expressed through the timing and intensity of GnRH secretion. The frequency of pulses and possibly their amplitude determine the amounts of LH and FSH and their ratio to each other. Too rapid a pulse frequency, such as three pulses per hour, causes suppression of both LH and FSH in an ovariectomized rhesus monkey model (Knobil, 1980). If, on the other hand, the pulse frequency of GnRH is delayed

Figure 1

Neuroanatomic relationship of noradrenergic, dopaminergic, beta endorphin, and GnRH neurons within the anterior hypothalamus.

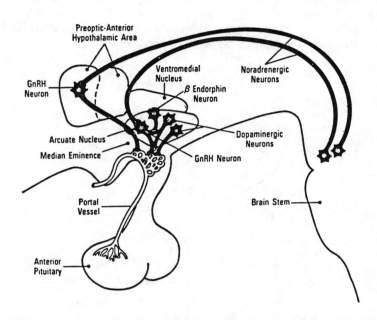

From "Neuroendocrine regulation of gonadotropin and prolactin secretion in women: Disorders in reproduction," by S.S.C. Yen, 1982. In J.L. Vaitukikaitis (Ed.), *Clinical reproductive neuroendocrinology*. New York: Elsevier Biomedical. Reprinted with permission.

to one pulse every 3 hours, then FSH is secreted in much larger quantities in response to GnRH than is LH (see Figure 2). GnRH pulse frequency changes during the menstrual cycle with hourly pulses during the follicular and less frequent ones during the luteal phase. It may be that the control of the timing of these pulses determines hormonal events of the menstrual cycle.

The arcuate nucleus, main site of GnRH production, sits in the center of the medial basal hypothalamus where numerous neurotransmitter neurons in close proximity may influence its secretion (see Figure 1). GnRH appears to be under complex positive and negative control. Norepinephrine may be a major stimulator of GnRH in the primate (Bhattacharya, Dierchshke, Yamaji, & Knobil, 1972), although its role is less clear in men than in the rat.

GnRH secretion may be suppressed by at least two neurotransmitters. Both beta endorphin and dopamine are closely related anatomically to the GnRH neuron in the hypothalamus. Both appear to have negative effects on GnRH secretion. Because beta endorphin appears to stimulate dopamine, it may be

Figure 2

In the ovariectomized rhesus monkey with the arcuate nucleus of the hypothalamus ablated, the pulse frequency of exogenous GnRH determines the response of LH and FSH. At a pulse frequency of 6 mcg. per hour, LH response is higher, FSH response is lower. At a pulse frequency of 6 mcg. every three hours, the LH peak is relatively delayed and lower while the FSH peak is markedly enhanced as well as delayed.

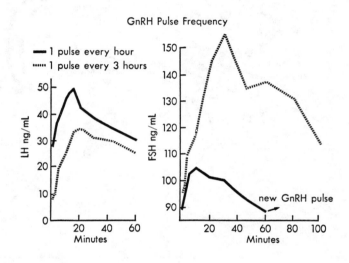

From "The Neuroendocrine control of the menstrual cycle," by E. Knobil, 1980, *Recent progress in hormone research*, **36**, p. 53. Reprinted with permission.

that endorphin suppression of GnRH acts mainly through dopamine (Yen, 1982) (see Figure 3). It is not clear whether these inhibitors act by changing the pulse frequency and/or by altering the amplitude of GnRH.

Evidence for the role of beta endorphin and dopamine in suppression of gonadotropin-releasing hormone comes from the use of specific receptor blockers or antagonists. Naloxone is a receptor blocker for endorphin (Quigley & Yen, 1980) and Metochlopramide is an antagonist for dopamine (Quigley, Judd, Gilliland, & Yen, 1979). Studies in which Naloxone was infused into normal women in various phases of the cycle showed an increase in LH during the luteal but not the early follicular phase (Quigley & Yen, 1980). These results suggest that endorphin plays an inhibitory role in the normal luteal phase. Direct infusion of beta endorphin in man or woman results in decreased

Figure 3

Diagrammatic illustration of postulated inhibitory relationship between beta endorphin and dopamine on gonadotropin releasing hormone (LRF) secretion within the anterior hypothalamus.

NEUROENDOCRINE REGULATION

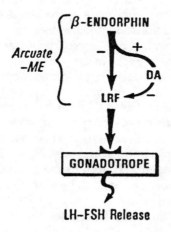

From "Neuroendocrine regulation of gonadotropin and prolactin secretion in women: Disorders in reproduction," by S.S.C. Yen, 1982. In J.L. Vaitukikaitis (Ed.), *Clinical reproductive neuroendocrinology*. New York: Elsevier Biomedical. Reprinted with permission.

LH levels and increased prolactin levels (Reid, Hoff, Yen, & Li, 1981). Both endorphin effects appear to be acting at the hypothalamic level.

The ovarian control of reproduction by feedback on GnRH is not clearly worked out. Although it is apparent from the work of Knobil (1980) that the major feedback occurs at the level of the pituitary gland, hypothalamic estrogen infusion will inhibit gonadotropin-releasing hormone directly (Chappel, Reskar, Norman, & Spies, 1981). In humans, progesterone probably acts as a suppressor of GnRH secretion at a hypothalamic level, perhaps by reducing the frequency of gonadotropin discharges (Knobil, 1980). Estrogen may have part of its hypothalamic effect through its conversion into the strange molecular blend of estrogen with a catecholamine side chain, catecholestrogens. Catecholestrogens appear to compete for enzymes required in the production of dopamine and norepinephrine in the hypothalamus (Lloyd & Weisz, 1978).

Pituitary Gonadotropins

Reproduction, initiated by the hypothalamus, is effected through two pituitary hormones. The gonadotropins, LH and FSH, are produced by the same cell, and are controlled by the same stimulating hormone, GnRH. They are found only within the anterior pituitary. Gonadotropins share an identical alpha chain with thyroid stimulating hormone and with human chorionic gonadotropin (hCG), which is normally made by the uterus and present only during pregnancy. LH and FSH are under the positive stimulatory control of gonadotropin-releasing hormone. In the absence of hypothalamic stimulation, LH and FSH both decrease to very low levels.

The pituitary has two apparent "pools" for the gonadotropins, a pool which can be initially released with a bolus of gonadotropin-releasing hormone and a pool which is in reserve for later release (Hof, Lasley, Wang, & Yen, 1977). Gonadotropin-releasing hormone causes the synthesis, storage, activation, and release of LH and FSH. The differential control of LH versus FSH levels seems to be through the frequency of GnRH pulses (see Figure 2).

Pituitary gonadotropins are regulated from below as well as from above. LH and FSH release are under feedback control by the major gonadal steroids, estrogen, and progesterone (see Figure 4). Estrogen, when at low levels, has a negative feedback effect and increases the synthesis and storage of FSH and LH. It does not appear to alter LH secretion but inhibits FSH secretion. During the middle of the cycle when the hormonal explosion takes place, estrogen maintains a high level which stimulates a sustained pulse of FSH and LH (commonly termed *surge*). Estrogen feedback has become positive rather than negative (Knobil, 1980).

Progesterone also controls LH and FSH secretion. Progesterone administration in normal and hypogonadal women pretreated with estrogen is necessary for a midcycle surge of normal intensity and duration (Lui & Yen, 1983). The elegant work of Knobil and colleagues (1980) has shown that ovarian steroids determine the midcycle surge. In the monkey model the hypothalamus was blocked from any feedback, yet the huge surge of LH and FSH still occurred. Thus the hypothalamus plays only a permissive role in the dramatic events in the middle of the menstrual cycle.

The Ovary

Mysterious, largely unnoticed events happen within the ovary during every cycle. A recent review summarized the current understanding of folliculogenesis (Fritz & Speroff, 1982). The first event is recruitment of follicles. Of the thousands of potential egg-containing follicles which rest quietly through

Figure 4

The neuroendocrine and gonadal feedback control of gonadotropin and GnRH secretion.

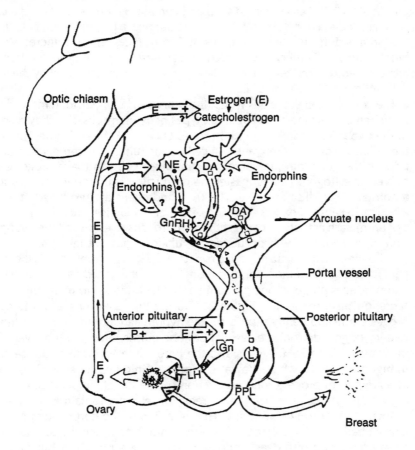

From "Asymmetrical ovarian function during recruitment and selection of the dominant follicle in the menstrual cycle of a rhesus monkey," by G.S. diZerega, E.L. Marut, C.K. Turner, and G.D. Hodgen, 1980, *Journal of Clinical Endocrinology and Metabolism*, **51**, p. 698. Reprinted with permission.

most of the ovarian life cycle, several are recruited and begin to grow. One of the responsive follicles stimulated during the early follicular phase becomes dominant. It has the most hormone-producing cells and becomes the controlling part of the ovary from about Day 8 for the rest of that cycle. The dominant follicle, which will release the prepared ovum, controls the timing of the midcycle surge of gonadotropins by its production of estradiol and preovulatory production of progesterone (diZerega, Marut, Turner, & Hodgen, 1980; Lui & Yen, 1983; McNatty, Smith, Makris, Osathanondh, & Ryan, 1979).

At birth the ovaries contain all the germ cells (ova) they will ever have. The ovaries are in a resting state. The primordial follicle is extremely small (approximately 15 micrometers in size) and contains granulosa cells and a clear zone around the oocyte. Early in the follicular phase the granulosa cell, under the stimulation of FSH, increases its own receptor and increases the biochemical machinery with which to make estrogen out of the androgens, androstenedione and testosterone. These androgens are produced by the theca cell under the influence of LH.

The complicated processes within the ovary can be understood more clearly if one remembers there are two main types of ovarian cells, and they respond to the two main gonadotropin hormones LH and FSH (see Figure 5). Under the influence of FSH, the granulosa cell can acquire LH receptors so that just prior to the gonadotropin surge, the granulosa cell can make progesterone as well as estrogen. This progesterone production is important in producing a normal surge (diZerega et al., 1980). If androgens are produced in excess amounts because of excess secretion of LH, or if there is inadequate granulosa cell aromatase activity to convert these androgens to estradiol, then suppression of follicular growth occurs and ovulation does not take place.

Following the dramatic midcycle events of the gonadotropin surge, the dominant follicle has become luteinized (from then on it is called the corpus luteum) and produces progesterone predominantly. It continues to maintain a lower secretion of estrogen (see Figure 6). During the luteal phase of the cycle, progesterone apparently suppresses the hypothalamus and decreases the frequency of gonadotropin-releasing hormone pulses, lowering the level of LH in relationship to FSH. This is also the time when endorphins are secreted in higher amounts, which may also suppress GnRH (Quigley & Yen, 1980). The amount of progesterone production by the follicle appears to be determined by follicular growth and receptor number obtained during the preovulatory or follicular phase. The usual life of the corpus luteum is circumscribed, only 10 to 16 days. The mechanisms by which the corpus luteum stops production of progesterone and estrogen are not clear, but they may involve some luteolytic action of estrogen and perhaps some effect of prolactin.

Clinical Evaluation of the Menstrual Cycle

The mechanisms that we have just reviewed usually present themselves very simply as menstrual flow and are caused by withdrawal of progesterone and estrogen from the endometrium in the uterus. The first few days of the follicular phase may be dominated by lower abdominal cramping, back pain, and general malaise secondary to prostaglandin production by the uterus. The

Figure 5

Diagrammatic representation of ovarian cells, their response to gonadotropins and hormonal production.

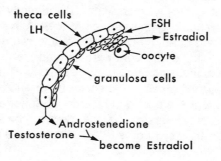

Figure 6

Ovarian cellular response to gonadotropin and hormone production within the follicle. The temporal relationship of gonadotropin and ovarian steroid secretion in the normal menstrual cycle.

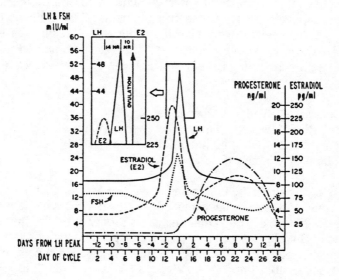

From "Asymmetrical ovarian function during recruitment and selection of the dominant follicle in the menstrual cycle of a rhesus monkey," by G.S. diZerega, E.L. Marut, C.K. Turner, and G.D. Hodgen, 1980, *Journal of Clinical Endocrinology and Metabolism*, **51**, p. 698. Reprinted with permission.

follicular phase, after the end of flow, is rather quiet. It may be ended by mild unilateral lower abdominal pain lasting a few hours occurring at the time of follicular rupture and ovulation. An increase in cervical mucus that is clear and stringy indicates the high-estrogen levels at midcycle.

The end of the follicular phase and the beginning of the luteal phase is difficult to document clinically. It is signalled indirectly by the rise in basal temperature, which marks progesterone production by the corpus luteum. If serial ultrasounds are done, an ovulatory follicle can usually be visualized which will attain a size of 2.0 cm or greater and then shrink following egg release. The luteal phase usually lasts 10 to 16 days. This is the phase during which most ovulatory women experience one or another of the symptoms termed molimina, which are mild but include dysphoria, fluid retention, appetite change, and breast tenderness. If these symptoms are severe they are termed the premenstrual syndrome (PMS). The onset of menstrual flow ends the luteal phase.

Adaptations of Reproduction

The hormonal mechanisms that have been reviewed have only briefly outlined some of the complexities involved. Subsequent chapters will discuss the endocrine changes which occur with exercise and athletic training. The best hypothesis that seems to fit what we understand of these mechanisms is that the adaptive reponses to exercise are mediated by the hypothalamus (Prior, 1982). In order to understand the changes that occur with exercise, a series of hypotheses about possible mechanisms can be proposed and tested. Four of these mechanisms/challenges which can alter reproductive activity might be

1. nutritional deprivation (Warren, 1983);
2. psychic threat (Warren, Siris, & Petrovich, 1976);
3. systemic illness (Fries, Nillims, & Pettersson, 1974); and
4. conditioning exercise (Prior, 1982).

Because of the similarity in responses, we can assume that the pattern of hypothalamic and menstrual cycle change associated with all types of challenge is the same. The actual change is probably in the timing and/or amplitude of GnRH pulsation. If the changes are an adaptation to a particular kind of challenge, then we can hypothesize, as has been shown, that these changes are reversible (Prior, Pride, Vigna, & Ho Yuen, 1983; Prior, Ho Yuen, Clement, Bowie, & Thomas, 1982). Because the adaptive changes develop to prevent pregnancy, when pregnancy does occur the fetus would be relatively protected. Preliminary evidence suggests this is true.

Summary

Amazing events happen every menstrual cycle. These events are under finely tuned control, responsive to external environmental influences, and allow the reproductive system to adapt. Details of the hormonal changes during the menstrual cycle and how these hormones adapt to acute and chronic exericse are not clearly understood at present. However, an understanding of the normal menstrual cycle is essential before the special situation of the menstrual cycle and exercise can be studied adequately.

References

Bhattacharya, A.N., Diercshke, V.J., Yamaji, T., & Knobil, E. (1972). The pharmacologic blockade of the circhoral mode of LH secetion in the ovariectomized rhesus monkey. *Endocrinology*, **90**, 778-786.

Boyer, R.M. (1978). Control of the onset of puberty. *Annual Review of Medicine*, **29**, 509-520.

Chappel, S.C., Reskar, J.A., Norman, R.L., & Spies, H.G. (1981). Studies in rhesus monkeys on the site where estrogen inhibits gonadotropins: Delivery of 17 beta estradiol to the hypothalamus and pituitary gland. *Journal of Clinical Endocrinology and Metabolism*, **51**, 1-8.

Crowley, W.F., & McArthur, J.W. (1980). Stimulation of the normal menstrual cycle in Kallmann's syndrome by pulsatile administration of luteinizing hormone releasing hormone (LHRH). *Journal of Clinical Endocrinology and Metabolism*, **51**, 173-179.

diZerega, G.S., Marut, E.L., Turner, C.K., & Hodgen, G.D. (1980). Asymmetrical ovarian function during recruitment and selection of the dominant follicle in the menstrual cycle of a rhesus monkey. *Journal of Clinical Endocrinology and Metabolism*, **51**, 698-701.

Elkind-Hirsch, K., Ravinkar, V., Shift, I., Tulchinsky, D., & Ryan, K.J. (1982). Determination of endogenous immunoreactive luteinizing hormone releasing hormone in human plasma. *Journal of Clinical Endocrinology and Metabolism*, **54**, 602-607.

Fries, H., Nillims, S.J., & Pettersson, F. (1974). Epidemiology of secondary amenorrhea. *American Journal of Obstetrics and Gynecology*, **118**, 473-479.

Fritz, M.A., & Speroff, L. (1982). The endocrinology of the menstrual cycle: The interaction of the folliculo-genesis and neuroendocrine mechanisms. *Fertility and Sterility*, **38**, 509-529.

Hoff, J.D., Lasley, B.L., Wang, C.S., & Yen, S.S.C. (1977). Regulation during the menstrual cycle. *Journal of Clinical Endocrinology and Metabolism*, **44**, 302-312.

Knobil, E. (1980). The neuroendocrine control of the menstrual cycle. *Recent Progress in Hormone Research*, **36**, 53-88.

Lui, J.H., & Yen, S.S.C. (1983). Induction of mid-cycle gonadotropin surge by ovarian steroids in women: A critical evaluation. *Journal of Clinical Endocrinology and Metabolism*, **57**, 797-802.

Lloyd, T., & Weisz, J. (1978). Direct inhibition of tyrosine hydroxylase activity by catecholestrogens. *Journal of Biological Chemistry*, **253**, 4841-4845.

Marshall, J.C., & Kelch, R.P. (1979). Low-dose pulsatile gonadotropin releasing hormone in anorexia nervosa: A model of human pubertal development. *Journal of Clinical Endocrinology and Metabolism*, **49**, 712-718.

McNatty, K.D., Smith, D.M., Makris, A., Osathanondh, R., & Ryan, K.H. (1979). The micro-environment of the human antral follicle. *Journal of Clinical Endocrinology and Metabolism*, **49**, 851-860.

Prior, J.C. (1982). Endocrine "conditioning" with endurance training: A preliminary review. *Canadian Journal of Applied Sport Sciences*, **7**, 148-157.

Prior, J.C., Ho Yuen, B., Clement, P., Bowie, L., & Thomas, J. (1982). Reversible luteal phase changes and infertility associated with marathon training. *Lancet*, **1**, 269-270.

Prior, J.C., Pride, S.D., Vigna, Y., & Ho Yuen, B. (1983). The marathon and reversible luteal phase shortening: A controlled prospective study. Abstract. *Medicine and Science in Sport and Exercise*, **15**, 174.

Quigley, M.E., Judd, S.J., Gilliland, G.B., & Yen, S.S.C. (1979). The effects of a dopamine antagonist on the release of gonadotropin and prolactin in normal women and women with hyperprolactinemic anovulation. *Journal of Clinical Endocrinology and Metabolism*, **48**, 718-720.

Quigley, M.E., & Yen, S.S.C. (1980). The role of endogenous opiates on LH secretion during the menstrual cycle. *Journal of Clinical Endocrinology and Metabolism*, **51**, 179-180.

Reid, R.L., Hof, J.D., Yen, S.S.C., & Li, C.H. (1981). Effects of exogenous beta endorphin on pituitary hormone secretion and its disappearance rate in normal human subjects. *Journal of Clinical Endocrinology and Metabolism*, **52**, 1179-1184.

Schally, A.V., Arimura, A., & Kastin, A.J. (1973). Hypothalamic regulatory hormones. *Science*, **179**, 341-350.

Warren, M.P. (1983). Effects of undernutrition of reproductive function in the human. *Endocrine Reviews*, **4**, 363-377.

Warren, M., Siris, E., & Petrovich, C. (1976). The influence of severe illness on gonadotropin secretion in the post-menopausal female. *Journal of Clinical Endocrinology and Metabolism*, **45**, 99-104.

Yen, S.S.C. (1982). Neuroendocrine regulation of gonadotropin and prolactin secretion in women: Disorders in reproduction. In J.L. Vaitukikaitis (Ed.), *Clinical reproductive neuroendocrinology* (pp. 137-174). New York: Elsevier Biomedical.

Reactions to Jerilynn Prior's Presentation

Reactor: Janet Hall

In looking at the spectrum of menstrual cycle changes and their causes, we have to consider that it includes women who stopped having cycles, women who have less frequent cycles, women who have short luteal phases, and women who may have no observable changes. There have been astounding advances in the understanding of the control of reproduction over the last 10 years, and the amount of information is accumulating exponentially. What does exercise do that interferes with neuroendocrine control of reproductive function? How do body weight and weight loss fit into this scheme of things? We also have to remember that there are other things besides exercise that can result in menstrual changes—things like pregnancy, premature ovarian failure (whether of genetic or idiopathic origin), alterations in thyroid function, hyperprolactinemia, and polycystic ovaries. Dr. Prior, you mentioned the hypothesis that the changes were occurring in the hypothalamus. Would you comment further?

Discussion

Jerilynn Prior: My hypothesis is that the changes are happening in the hypothalamus. I would bet that it is the pulse frequency of GnRH which is altered and that the pulse frequency is altered not only by endorphins but also by factors we are not familiar with yet. The common key between exercise, illness, psychic stress, undernutrition, and nutritional changes is not clear but I would guess that it probably has something to do with insulin receptor sensitivity in the hypothalamus.

Edwin Dale: Your comments about anthropology were very intriguing. The stress of just running may be no different from the saber-toothed tiger at the door of the cave ten thousand years ago or the stress of having to go out and be a hunter/gatherer. We have tried to look at the so-called stress hormones and have measured catecholamines, catecholestrogens, and beta-endorphins and catecholamines are elevated. We postulate that these shut off both LHRH (LRF) and GnRH, which when shut off would reduce LH, leading to the inhibition of ovulation and the development of the follicle. So stress does have a role. We need to measure it and quantify it. I would think that the catecholestrogens may be one of the causes.

Barbara Drinkwater: In light of the criticisms of using basal body temperature (BBT), do you feel BBT adequately represents luteal phase length and is it possible to use that rather than a complete endocrine profile?

Jerilynn Prior: I devised a form that was actually just a list for recording temperature. I don't have the subjects do any plotting, so that eliminates one source of error. Women determine their oral temperature from a celsius thermometer so that the numbers are spread apart and you can reliably read a tenth of a degree. We plot the results across the graph. I have used the quantitative method that Volman used and determine an arithmetic mean from all those temperatures. The time (place) on the graph where the mean crosses the actual temperature curve is called an intercept. Volman says that one side of the intercept is the premenstrual phase and the other is the postmenstrual phase. In terms of clinical experience, it correlates closely enough with luteal and follicular phases. If a person has scanty data we simply don't analyze it. The database I've used (Volman) is from 691 women, 31,645 BBTs including various gynecological ages (from ages 11 to 65), normal men, and women on oral contraceptives as controls. Because of the cost of hormone assays, I think that basal body temperature can be used as an alternative because it can be looked at in a quantitative way that is reproducible and it has a good population base.

Unknown: Is there any correlation between the rise in BBT and progesterone levels?

Edwin Dale: There was a study where they looked at basal body temperature and LH and the short luteal phase. The BBTs were not particularly good.

Jerilynn Prior: Yes, but they didn't use the same method of BBT recording.

Arend Bonen: In the study with Bowman in 1981 where they looked at records and tried to correlate with LH levels throughout the menstrual cycle, the BBT records were not particularly good indicators of the LH peak day. I think we can't ignore that kind of data.

Jerilynn Prior: We have to ignore it because the physicians looking at it were not looking at it in a quantitative way. They were looking at it as they do in an infertility clinic where you eyeball the data.

Arend Bonen: I don't disagree, but I think we ought to examine the use of BBTs critically. It is easy for those doing some of the hormonal data to also do BBT data with it. But we have to be a little careful with just using BBTs now.

Jerilynn Prior: But it doesn't matter when LH peaks. It matters to me that the rise in BBT occurs up until the next day of menses.

Charlotte Sanborn: Yes, BBT works, maybe with infertile women. I tried BBTs in 1978 in a training study with 40 athletic college women. There was no way you could determine if it was biphasic. The only ones who were found biphasic were the athletes who wanted to become pregnant.

Jerilynn Prior: Most people don't know how to plot accurately and I think it makes the difference between reliable and unreliable data.

Michelle Warren: I get challenged like this by scientists who are used to measuring levels and getting exact numbers. But unfortunately we are not dealing with an exact phenomenon. It would be a shame if we all stopped doing basal body temperatues. It gives us an idea of what is going on over a 30-, 60-, or 90-day period that sampling at any one time cannot do. Preliminary data indicate that athletes don't have normal basal temperatures, which in itself is very interesting. So when you see something that looks bizarre, don't throw it out because in itself it may be significant.

Elizabeth Miescher: At CSU, we do a saliva/progesterone test (not published). The women spit in the morning at the same time each day after they have brushed their teeth (preferably) and then we assay the samples for progesterone. The cost for this assay is minimal (less than $3 per sample) if you do your own work and you develop your own reagents. It is not hard to do and it gives a sample that is correlated with blood levels. It lets you determine the rise in progesterone and the magnitude of rise. It is simple, takes away the possibility of making mistakes on basal body temperature, and eliminates some of the discrepancies. It is used commonly in pediatrics. The order of magnitude is 10 times less than progesterone levels in the blood; it is a reflection of what is going on in the blood, but the blood is better. You need to accept the deficiencies of the method if you use it.

Barbara Drinkwater: I second Arend Bonen's comment here that if you have the opportunity to do full endocrine profiles, also take BBTs and let those of us who do not have access to the mint hear from you about how well they correspond.

Marilyn Morehead: How do you go about measuring beta endorphin levels, because beta endorphin levels at the hypothalamic level would be quite different from what you would find in other areas. What are the possibilities of using other aspects of the macromolecule?

Janet Hall: We are not going to sample from the hypothalamus. But we are now working on using a blocker.

6

Endocrine Alterations
With Exercise and Training

Arend Bonen
Dalhousie University

There is now widespread recognition that alterations in menstrual function occur during periods of intense training. Much of this information has been derived from surveys of athletes (Feicht, Johnson, Martin, Sparks, & Wagner, 1978; Feicht-Sanborn, Martin, & Wagner, 1982; Lutter & Cushman, 1982; Shangold & Levine, 1982; Speroff & Redwine, 1980; Webb, Millan, & Stoltz, 1979; Zaharieva, 1965) with a focus toward chronicling the incidence of secondary amenorrhea. From such studies, several predisposing factors have appeared consistently, namely, the young age of the athlete, training prior to menarche, training distance (runners), and training history (i.e., number of years) (for review see Bonen, 1983; Bonen & Keizer, 1984). Presumably, this is only a partial list of many possible predisposing factors.

The major limitation of the survey approach is that it dichotomizes women's menstrual cycles as being either normal or amenorrheic. Yet it is well known that normally menstruating women do not necessarily have a normal menstrual cycle; the inadequate (Ross & Hillier, 1978) and short luteal phase (diZerega & Hodgen, 1981; diZerega et al., 1981; Dodson, MacNaughton, & Coutts, 1975; Sherman & Korenman, 1974; Strott, Cargille, Ross, & Lipsett, 1970; Yoshida, Hattori, Suzuki, & Noda, 1979) menstrual cycles are two examples. Thus, our estimates of incidence of menstrual cycle irregularities in athletes

Studies from A. Bonen's laboratory are supported by Health and Welfare, Canada.

that are based on survey data are conservative at best (Bonen, 1985; Bonen & Keizer, 1981; Prior, Cameron, Yuen, & Thomas, 1982).

The menstrual cycle is under complex endocrine control (see Prior in chapter 5). Any disturbance in this cycle must therefore be caused by alterations in the endocrine milieu. Thus, it is necessary to study the known menstrual endocrine regulators before attempting to define the various anomalous menstrual functions of athletes.

Hormonal Responses to Exercise

Laboratory Studies

Because there are menstrual changes associated with heavy training, it is logical to assess the effects of exercise on the gonadotropin and ovarian hormones during exercise. Work from three laboratories (Bonen et al., 1979; Bonen et al., 1983; Jurkowski, Jones, Walker, Younglai, & Sutton, 1978; Keizer, 1983) has detailed a relatively consistent picture of ovarian and gonadotropic hormonal responses to exercise (see Table 1). Generally E_2 and P increase

Table 1

Summary of Gonadotropin and Ovarian Steroid Responses
to Acute Exercise in Untrained, Normally Menstruating Women

Hormone	Follicular phase			Luteal phase		
	Jurkowski	Keizer	Bonen	Jurkowski	Keizer	Bonen
LH	→↑[a]	↓	→	↓	↓	→
FSH	→↑[a]	→	→	→	→	→
Prolactin	—	↑	—	—	↑	—
E_2	↑[a]	↑		↑	↑	↑
P	→	↑[b]	→	↑	↑	↑

Data from Jurkowski et al. (1978); Keizer (1983); Bonen et al. (1979, 1983)
[a]at exhaustion only
[b]appears to be due to more sensitive assay

during exercise in the luteal phase with little or no change in P in the follicular phase except at the end of very heavy workloads. Absolute E_2 increments in the follicular phase are less than in the luteal phase (Jurkowski, 1978), though relative percent differences are similar in both phases (Keizer, 1983). Convincing evidence from Keizer's work (Keizer, Poortman, & Bunnik, 1980, 1981; Keizer, van Schaik, de Beer, Schiereck, & van Heeswijk, 1981) suggests that these increments are due to a decreased clearance of the ovarian steroids during exercise and for at least 30 min after exercise. Thus, it is unlikely that ovarian secretion of the hormones is enhanced.

The gonadotropin responses to exercise are variable. LH has been reported not to change (Bonen, Belcastro, Ling, & Simpson, 1981; Bonen et al., 1979; Jurkowski et al., 1978), but examination of some of the Jurkowski et al. data suggests that LH concentrations decrease in the luteal phase, a phenomenon also reported elsewhere (Keizer, 1983). In the follicular phase, both an increase and decrease have been reported in the same studies (Jurkowski et al., 1978; Keizer, 1983). FSH levels usually remain unchanged in the follicular and luteal phases during exercise. Prolactin levels increase differently depending on the degree of training (Brisson, Volle, Decarufel, Desharnais, & Tanaka, 1980; Keizer, 1983).

A pertinent question is whether the hormonal responses to exercise in untrained women provide an adequate picture of the responses that occur in trained women. The only available comprehensive report to date has been provided by Keizer (1983), who compared untrained women and marathon runners. Although the exercise protocols were somewhat different, they were comparable enough to provide meaningful comparisons (see Table 2). It was

Table 2

Comparisons of Hormonal Responses to Exercise in Untrained and Trained (Marathon) Women

Hormone	Follicular phase			Luteal phase		
	Untrained	Trained	U vs T	Untrained	Trained	U vs T
LH	↓	↓	NS	↓[a]	↓	NS
FSH	→	→	NS	→	→	NS
Prolactin	↑	↑	P < .05	(No data)	↑	—
E_2	↑	↑	NS	↑	↑	NS
P	↑	↑	NS	↑[a]	↑[b]	NS

[a]L vs F (%), P < .05
[b]F vs L (%), NS

evident from the data that the E_2 and P responses are more or less similar in the two groups, though the relative increase in P in the untrained women is greater in the luteal phases; no such phase effects for P increase occurred in the trained women. The percent LH decrease was more marked in the luteal phase of the untrained women, though a decrease of this gonadotropin occurred in both groups. Most notable, however, in this and other studies (e.g., Brisson et al., 1980) is the pronounced increase in prolactin that occurs in the trained woman compared to her untrained cohort. One might surmise that if this increase is provoked persistently during training bouts, an inhibiting effect on LH and FSH may result.

It should be remembered that the exercise periods used in laboratory studies frequently are shorter and at times less intense than those experienced during normal training schedules. Notwithstanding this limitation, the hormonal responses provoked by exercise of 60 to 90 min duration appear to be similar in untrained and trained women with the exception of prolactin.

Nonlaboratory Studies

It is difficult to obtain physiological data during competitive events such as the marathon for obvious reasons. Hale, Kosasa, Krieger, and Pepper (1983) have reported increment in prolactin (+327%) and FSH (+13.7%) and an LH decrement (−36.6%) after a marathon run. However, it is difficult to interpret their results because (a) control blood samples were obtained 7 to 10 days prior to the marathon, (b) the phase of the menstrual cycle of the subjects was not known, and (c) the hormone concentrations were not corrected for hemoconcentration (3 to 34%).

We have monitored hormone concentrations during a marathon by obtaining blood samples prior to, during, and after the marathon run. Responses for one of the subjects are shown in Figure 1. It is obvious from these data that the FSH levels were not markedly altered. The steroids (P, testosterone, DHEAS) increased during the run and remained elevated for at least 2 hours after the run.

Postexercise Effects

There are good reasons to examine the hormonal effects that remain after bouts of exercise. The sustained steroid responses after exercise may reflect prolonged metabolic clearance depression or enhanced ovarian and/or adrenal secretion. Whichever mechanism is prevalent, these steroid elevations may begin to inhibit the gonadotropins. While such inhibition was not evident in our study, it has been shown (Casper et al., unpublished data) that isoproterenol infusion (a B-adrenergic agonist that causes an increased MCR through the liver and kidney) reduces P and E_2 during a 5-hour period; it was

Figure 1

Hormonal responses before, during, and after a competitive marathon run in one subject.

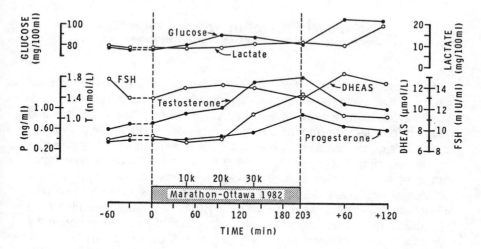

only near the end of a 4-hour observation period that an increase in LH became apparent. This suggests strongly that the steroid-induced alterations in gonadotropins take considerable time to manifest themselves and that the period of observation must extend beyond the time (i.e., ≤ 90 min) used in many studies.

We recently compared the gonadotropin responses in the follicular phase (Days 8 to 11) 2 hr before and after exercise to exhaustion (60 to 90 min) by sampling every 15 min throughout the experiment. LH levels generally increased in the postexercise period (Keizer & Bonen, 1983). There were marked individual differences among subjects, indicating that the postexercise observation period may still have been too brief.

Summary

The remaining problem with the acute exercise studies is that none have yet begun to reveal what factor(s) trigger the persistent gonadotropin alterations that have been reported in athletes (see below). Furthermore, while untrained and trained normally menstruating subjects appear to respond similarly to exercise (except for prolactin), the responses of individuals with short luteal phases and amenorrhea have yet to be documented. However, the hormonal effects that persist for some time after daily chronic exercise (i.e., training bouts) may ultimately be more significant than the transient hormonal responses during exercise.

Hormonal Profiles of Trained Women

The hormonal patterns of trained women throughout a normal or nonnormal menstrual cycle have not been thoroughly characterized. In some instances blood samples have been obtained on one or two occasions and analyzed for selected hormones. As noted previously (Bonen, in press), this approach is quite limiting as it presumes that infrequent sampling provides a correct description of any given hormone at any time and ignores the pulsatile pattern of some hormones. This limitation lessens the chance of finding statistically significant differences in hormone levels between normally menstruating women and athletes with menstrual anomalies. In studies from this laboratory we have relied on daily blood sampling to characterize the menstrual cycle (Bonen et al., 1981; Jacobson & Bonen, 1981; Jacobson, Wilkinson, & Bonen, 1983). The limitation of this method is that the pulsatile nature of gonadotropins is ignored, but the advantage is that repetitive measures that can be used to characterize the menstrual cycle are obtained. Several patterns have emerged from these studies and are discussed below according to the menstrual anomaly under consideration.

Normally Menstruating Athletes

Currently there is only one study (Keizer, 1983) comparing hormonal patterns in nonathletes and athletes who have normal menstrual cycles according to standard endocrine and gynecologic criteria. In this study, only the E_2 concentration in the follicular phase was markedly greater in the trained athletes. The high luteal phase LH levels in the untrained group seem unusual, as LH concentrations are usually reduced in the luteal phase (Bonen et al., 1979; Jurkowski et al., 1978) and were reduced in the athletes (see Table 3).

Amenorrheic Athletes

A few reports (Baker, Mathur, Kirk, & Williamson, 1981; Cumming, Strich, & Brumsting, 1981; Dale, Gerlach, & Wilhite, 1979; MacArthur et al., 1980; Shangold, Freeman, Thyson, & Gatz, 1979) have monitored blood samples in amenorrheic runners and contrasted these with observations in normally

Table 3

Comparison of Selected Hormones at Rest in Normally
Menstruating Untrained and Trained (Marathon) Subjects (M ± SEM)[a]

| Hormone | Untrained | | Trained | |
	Follicular phase	Luteal phase	Follicular phase	Luteal phase
LH (IU/ml)	9.0 ±0.6	11.0 ±1.5	9.4 ±0.2	5.8[b] ±1.1
FSH (IU/ml)	4.9 ±0.4	3.5 ±0.5	4.3 ±0.5	2.7 ±0.6
Prolactin (IU/ml)	0.34 ±0.10	0.27 ±0.02	0.22 ±0.05	0.21 ±0.06
E_2 (nmol/L)	0.15 ±0.03	0.56 ±0.07	0.56[b] ±0.12	0.44 ±0.03
P (nmol/L)	5.2 ±0.4	27.3 ±5.2	3.9 ±0.6	39.6 ±11.5

[a]Data from Keizer (1985). Reprinted with permission of the author.
[b]Follicular versus luteal $p < .05$

menstruating nonathletes or runners. (Whether these runners were indeed normally menstruating was not objectively assessed but assumed, based on self-reported incidence of regular menstrual bleeding.) In Baker et al., the concentrations of LH, FSH, P, E_2, and prolactin at rest did not differ statistically between groups. Others (Dale et al., MacArthur et al., Shangold et al.) have shown that LH levels are lower in amenorrheic runners and that based on the E1:E2 ratio, exercise amenorrhea differs from hypothalamic amenorrhea (Shangold et al.). However, hormones do fluctuate in amenorrheic women (Wu & Mikhail, 1979), making infrequent or irregular sampling unlikely to detect statistically significant differences.

More recent studies have shown that in amenorrheic runners the pulsatile activity of LH is much reduced in a 24-hour period. However, such athletes show an enhanced sensitivity to GnRH, suggesting that the pituitary can function appropriately (Wakat & Rogol, personal communication). Such pituitary hypersensitivity has also been observed elsewhere (MacArthur et al., 1980). Further details on the amenorrheic athlete can be found elsewhere in this volume (Feicht Sanborn, chapter 4).

Short Luteal Phase

The short luteal phase has been recognized since the early 1970s (Dodson et al., 1975; Sherman & Korenman, 1974; Strott et al., 1970). It is not detectable simply by monitoring the length of the menstrual cycle, which tends to be the same in normally menstruating women and those with a short luteal phase (Jacobson & Bonen, 1981; Jacobson et al., 1983) (see Figure 2). Although in athletes the short luteal phase has been reported via the use of basal body temperature records (Prior et al., 1982), endocrine data reveal that this is not a very reliable technique in short luteal phase cycles (Bonen & Keizer, 1984). The currently acceptable manner of detecting the short luteal phase is frequent sampling throughout the menstrual cycle so as to detect the day of the LH peak and the progession of the P concentration in the luteal phase.

Figure 2

Comparison of menstrual cycle length and the lengths of the follicular and luteal phase in mature, normally menstruating nonathletes and normally menstruating athletes. Note that data are based on daily LH measurements. This overtly "normal" menstrual cycle in the athletes is a short luteal phase ($P < 0.05$) cycle. (See also Table 4).

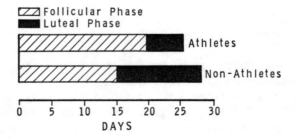

We have investigated daily hormone patterns in athletes with apparently normal menstrual cycles who were in fact experiencing short luteal phase cycles. This was first observed in young swimmers (Bonen et al., 1981) and more recently in older athletes (Jacobson et al., 1983) (see Table 4). Generally a short luteal phase occurred in all athletes. In the swimmers this was partly related to their young age but they still experienced shorter luteal phases than those of gynecologically age-matched teenagers. In the older athletes menstrual cycle length did not differ from normally menstruating nonathletes (see Figure 2).

Table 4

Comparisons of Durations of the Menstrual Cycle
and Its Phases in Athletes and Nonathletes ($M \pm$ SD)[a]

Group	Age (yrs)	Years beyond menarche	Menstrual cycle length (days)	Follicular phase (days)	Luteal phase (days)
Swimmers	15-19	2-4.5	20.0 ± 1.8[c,d]	14.5 ± 1.7	4.5 ± 0.6[c,d]
Teenagers	16-18	1-5	28.3 ± 6.4	20.0 ± 8.9	7.5 ± 3.0[c]
Adults	—	—	28.5 ± 3.4	16.0 ± 3.8[b]	13.4 ± 1.7[b]
Athletes	19-22	6-10	25.3 ± 4.5	19.0 ± 6.2	5.3 ± 2.1[e]
Nonathletes	21-29	9-15	28.5 ± 1.3	14.8 ± 1.5	12.8 ± 0.5

[a]Data from Bonen et al. (1981) and Jacobson, Wilkinson, and Bonen (1981).
[b]Data do not sum the menstrual cycle length as there are some missing data.
[c]$p < .05$ swimmers or teenagers versus adults
[d]$p < .05$ swimmers versus teenagers
[e]$p < .05$ athletes versus nonathletes

The hormonal profiles associated with short luteal phase cycles in swimmers are markedly different from those observed in the normal menstrual cycle (see Figure 3). Specifically, the major anomalies occurred in LH (elevated in follicular phase, $p < .05$) and FSH (depressed in follicular phase, $p < .05$) such that the FSH/LH ratio was far below normal (see Figure 4). These aberrant gonadotropin stimuli presumably provoked the subnormal development of the follicle, resulting in markedly reduced P concentrations in the luteal phase of swimmers' menstrual cycles.

In more recent studies with athletes 6 to 10 years beyond menarche, hormonal profiles are essentially similar to those profiles reported for younger swimmers (see Figure 5). Midfollicular, FSH ($P = .06$), and E_2 ($P = .05$) concentrations were lower in the athletes than in the nonathletes, and peak luteal phase P levels were lower in the athletes ($p < .05$) (Jacobson et al., 1983). One difference is that follicular phase LH levels were depressed in the older athletes ($p < .05$) while the young swimmers with a short luteal phase had elevated LH levels.

We have also had the opportunity to study two individual athletes on two occasions. The first participated in our initial experiments in 1975 (Bonen et al., 1981) and again in 1980 (Jacobson & Bonen, 1981). She was training on both occasions, at ages 15 and 21, respectively. On both occasions she

Figure 3

Comparison of selected hormones throughout the menstrual cycle of teenage swimmers. Grey shaded areas are $\bar{X} \pm$ ISD of normal menstruating cycles in adult women.

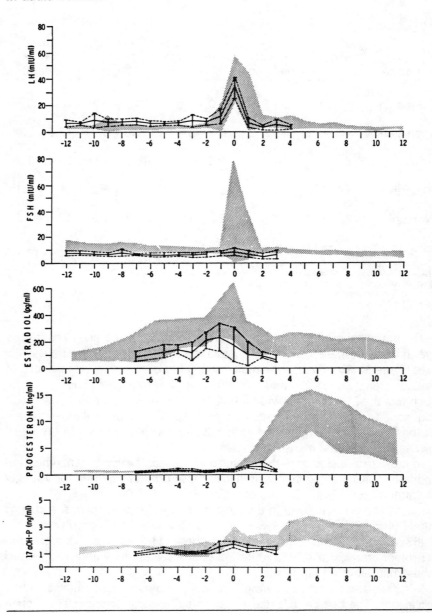

Figure 3 (Cont.)

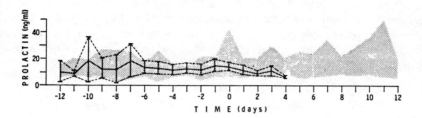

Figure 4

FSH/LH ratio in teenage swimmers (bottom) during the menstrual cycle and adult women (top). Grey shaded areas are $\overline{X} \pm$ ISD of normal menstrual cycle in adult women.

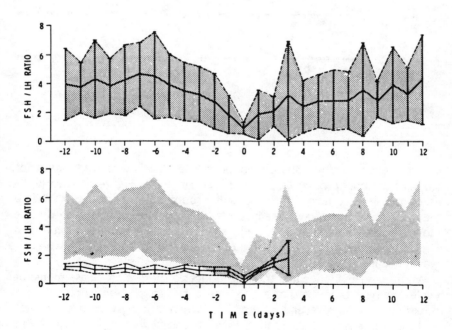

Figure 5

Comparison of selected hormones in a normally menstruating adult and an apparently normally menstruating adult athlete. Note the athlete has a short luteal phase cycle (see diminished P response in luteal phase). All athletes and nonathletes exhibited short luteal phase and normal cycles, respectively, in this study (data from Jacobson, Wilkinson, & Bonen, 1981).

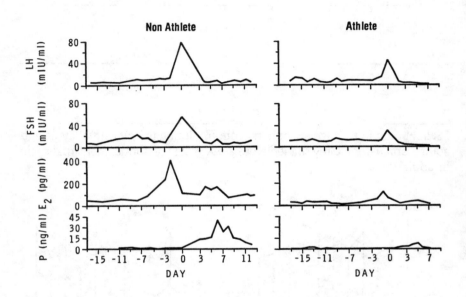

was also experiencing a short luteal phase menstrual cycle with remarkably similar hormonal profiles throughout each cycle (see Figure 6). Clearly, the luteal phase P concentration was still suboptimal ($\leqslant$ 3 ng/ml). Whether this individual has a chronically short luteal phase is difficult to discern. However, based on our data below, we believe that the training is implicated. Unfortunately, we were not able to obtain data for this individual when she was not training.

We do have evidence that training induces a short luteal phase menstrual cycle. We have monitored one swimmer in the second month of her training schedule and again several months later when training was more frequent and more intense in the month prior to the varsity championships. When training was moderate and infrequent (2 to 3 days/week) a normal cycle was observed (see Figure 7). With the intense training several months later, a short luteal phase cycle occurred. LH levels in this subject were elevated somewhat in the early follicular phase of her heavy training cycle, providing a reduced

FSH/LH ratio, or presumably an "anomalous" gonadotropin environment for the developing follicle. The result is again a markedly reduced P concentration.

The short luteal phases that we have documented to date exhibit hormonal profiles that are similar to those reported for nonathletic women with short luteal phases (Sherman & Korenman, 1974; Strott et al., 1970; Yoshida et al., 1979). This strongly suggests that this syndrome in athletes and nonathletes is caused by a similar mechanism. Apparently chronic training can provoke the onset of this process. Indeed data by Shangold (1979) based on one runner suggests that the degree of shortening of the luteal phase is proportional to weekly training mileage. Interestingly, all the athletes who think they have a normal menstrual cycle because of their regular menstrual periods always

Figure 6

Comparison of selected hormones throughout the menstrual cycle of a swimmer at age 15 and again at age 21. Note that a remarkably similar short luteal phase still existed. This individual was monitored during cycles that she was training.

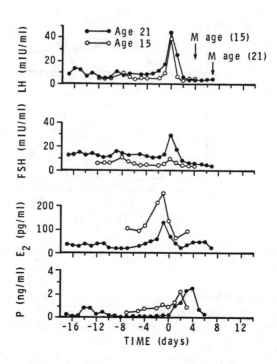

Figure 7

Comparison of selected hormones throughout the menstrual cycle in an athlete during moderate infrequent swim training and during very heavy frequent swim training. These two cycles are separated by one other menstrual cycle. Note the short luteal phase cycle during the heavy training period.

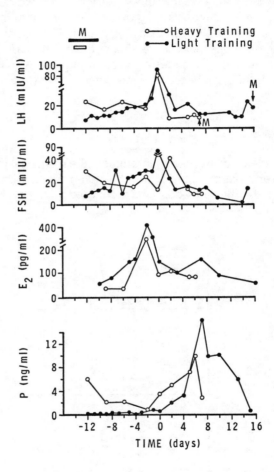

appear to have a short luteal phase, provided these data are obtained during a period of daily vigorous training.

The short luteal phase in subhuman primates has been induced via administration of inhibin-rich porcine follicular fluid (diZerega et al., 1981) or a long action GnRH agonist (Werlin & Hodgen, 1983). This yielded hormonal profile data that were remarkably similar to the data on our swimmers (Bonen et al., 1981). We therefore commenced studies to ascertain the presence of inhibin-like activity (ILA) in human sera obtained from athletes and nonathletes (see Table 4). Unfortunately, such differences were not apparent between the two groups, though we did observe ILA activity throughout the menstrual cycle (Jacobson et al., 1983).

Based on our studies, the short luteal phase cycle is difficult to detect but highly prevalent in athletes. Its overt appearance is remarkably like a normal menstrual cycle (i.e., normal length and menstruation). The mechanisms of onset of this cycle are not yet defined but likely attributable to deficient follicular phase gonadotropin levels. Recent evidence with subhuman primates implicates a possible hypothalamic dysfunction, i.e., a slowing of the frequency of GnRH pulse reduces FSH (Pohl, Richardson, Hutchinson, Germak, & Knobil, 1983). However, folliculogenesis is impaired even with normal FSH levels (Pohl et al., 1983).

Prospective Training Studies

As is evident by now, most of the available endocrine data have been based on comparisons between athletes and nonathletes. Few studies are available that have attempted to evaluate the endocrine alterations attributable to training. When studies were performed in this laboratory with very intense training, marked alterations in the menstrual cycle were provoked. The endocrine responses to a standard bout of exercise were investigated at the end of 8 to 11 weeks of training and were markedly reduced. However, as we noted in that report (Bonen et al., 1979) the uncertainty of the menstrual cycle phase at the posttraining retesting limits the interpretation of those results.

In the studies by Keizer (1983), a 3-month training program was undertaken. Comparisons of E_2, P, and prolactin responses to standardized exercise workloads before and after training in both the follicular and luteal phases did not provoke any changes in the relative responses. The menstrual cycle was apparently not altered by the training. The training intensity seemed lower than in our studies.

Women who volunteered to train for about 15 months to attempt to complete a marathon did experience alterations in their menstrual hormones (Boyden, Pamenter, Stanforth, Rotkis, & Wilmore, 1982). Interestingly, though, none of these subjects developed secondary amenorrhea. The onset of short luteal phases was apparently not investigated.

Summary

There is now no question that chronic exercise will alter the normal menstrual cycle. This can range from inducing secondary amenorrhea to more covert changes such as short luteal phase. However, one must also look beyond the exercise period to ascertain hormonal alterations that persist. Presumably these prolonged effects are ultimately more significant biologically and may provide a better indication as to the causes of exercise-induced menstrual irregularities. It is probably such studies that will provide further answers in this area of research, and which will bridge the gap between the acute, exercise-induced responses and the marked alterations in resting gonadotropin levels observed in highly trained athletes. In addition, studies are also required to establish whether the various menstrual anomalies observed in exercising women have the same mechanistic basis as similar anomalies in nonexercising women. Clearly such efforts require endocrine-based investigations. Concurrently, the mechanistic studies being performed with subhuman primates (e.g., diZerega & Hodgen, 1981; Pohl et al., 1983; Werlin & Hodgen, 1983) serve as extremely useful adjuncts to studies with athletic populations and provide data that we cannot ignore.

References

Baker, E.R., Mathur, R.S., Kirk, R.F., & Williamson, H.O. (1981). Female runners and secondary amenorrhea: Correlation with age, parity, mileage, and plasma hormonal and sex-hormone-binding glubulin concentrations. *Fertility and Sterility*, **36**, 183-187.

Bonen, A. (1983). Exercise-related disturbances in the menstrual cycle. In *Future directions in exercise biology*. Champaign, IL: Human Kinetics Publishers.

Bonen, A., Belcastro, A.N., Ling, W.Y., & Simpson, A.A. (1981). Profiles of selected hormones during menstrual cycles of teenage athletes. *Journal of Applied Physiology: Respiratory Environmental Exercise Physiology*, **50**, 545-551.

Bonen, A., Haynes, F., Watson-Wright, W., Sopper, M., Pierce, G., Low, M.P., & Graham, T.E. (1983). Effects of menstrual cycle on metabolic responses to exercise. *Journal of Applied Physiology: Respiratory Environmental Exercise Physiology*, **55**, 1506-1513.

Bonen, A., & Keizer, H.A. (1984). Athletic menstrual cycle irregularity (AMI): Endocrine responses to exercise and training. *The Physician and Sportsmedicine*, **12**, 78-94.

Bonen, A., Ling, W.Y., MacIntyre, K.P., Neil, R., McGrail, J.C., & Belcastro, A.N. (1979). Effects of exercise on the serum concentrations of FSH, LH, progesterone and estradiol. *European Journal of Applied Physiology for Occupational Physiology*, **42**, 15-23.

Boyden, T.W., Pamenter, R.W., Stanforth, P., Rotkis, T., & Wilmore, J.H. (1982). Evidence for mild thyroidal impairment in women undergoing endurance training. *Journal of Clinical Endocrinology and Metabolism*, **53**, 53-56.

Brisson, G.R., Volle, M.A., Decarufel, D., Desharnais, M., & Tanaka, M. (1980). Exercise-induced dissociation of the blood prolactin response in young women according to their sports habits. *Hormone and Metabolic Research*, **12**, 201-205.

Cumming, D.C., Strich, G., & Brumsting, L.A. (1981). Acute exercise related endocrine changes in women runners and nonrunners. *Fertility and Sterility*, **36**, 421-426.

Dale, E., Gerlach, D.H., & Wilhite, A.L. (1979). Menstrual dysfunction in distance runners. *Obstetrics and Gynecology*, **54**, 47-53.

Dodson, K.S., MacNaughton, M.C., & Coutts, J.R.T. (1975). Infertility in women with apparently ovulatory cycles: Vol. I. Comparison of their plasma sex steroid and gonadotropin profiles with those in the normal cycle. *British Journal of Obstetrics and Gynecology*, **82**, 615-624.

Feicht, C.B., Johnson, T.S., Martin, B.J., Sparks, K.E., & Wagner, W.W. (1978). Secondary amenorrhea in athletes. *Lancet*, **2**, 1145-1146.

Feicht-Sanborn, C., Martin, B.J., & Wagner, W.W. (1982). Is athletic amenorrhea specific to runners? *American Journal of Obstetrics and Gynecology*, **143**, 859-861.

Hale, R.W., Kosasa, T., Krieger, J., & Pepper, S. (1983). A marathon: The immediate effect on female runners' luteinizing hormone, follicle stimulating hormone, prolactin, testosterone and cortisol levels. *American Journal of Obstetrics and Gynecology*, **146**, 550-556.

Jacobson, W., & Bonen, A. (1981). Persistence of a short luteal phase in a young athlete after 5 years. *Canadian Journal of Applied Sport Sciences* (Abstract), **6**, 155.

Jacobson, W., Wilkinson, M., & Bonen, A. (1983). Inhibin like activity in serum from young female athletes with luteal phase defects. *Medicine and Science for Sport and Exercise*, **15**, 173.

Jurkowski, J.E., Jones, N.L., Walker, W.C., Younglai, E.V., & Sutton, J.R. (1978). Ovarian hormonal responses to exercise. *Journal of Applied Physiology: Respiratory Environmental Exercise Physiology*, **44**, 109-114.

Keizer, H.A. (1983). *Hormonal responses in women as a function of physical exercise and training.* Doctoral dissertation, Ryksuniversiteit Limburg, Maastricht, The Netherlands. Haarlem, The Netherlands: deVrieseborch.

Keizer, H.A., & Bonen, A. (1983, September). Post-exercise changes in gonadotropin secretion pattern in women. International Congress on Sports and Health, Maastricht, The Netherlands. *International Journal of Sports Medicine* (Abstract Service), p. 23.

Keizer, H.A., Poortman, J., & Bunnik, G.S.J. (1980). Influence of physical exercise on sex-hormone metabolism. *Journal of Applied Physiology*: REEP, **48**, 765-769.

Keizer, H.A., Poortman, J., & Bunnik, G.S.J. (1981). Influence of physical exercise on sex-hormone metabolism. In J. Poortman & G. Niset (Eds.), *Biochemistry of exercise* (pp. 229-236). Vol IV-B, International Series on Sport Sciences, IIB. Baltimore: University Park Press.

Keizer, H.A., van Schaik, F.W., de Beer, E.L., Schiereck, P., & van Heeswijk, G. (1981). Exercise-induced changes in estradiol metabolism and their possible physiological meaning. *Medicine and sport*, **14**, 125-140. Karger, Basel.

Lutter, J.M., & Cushman, S. (1982). Menstrual patterns in female runners. *The Physician and Sportsmedicine*, **10**(9), 60-72.

MacArthur, J.W., Buller, B.A., Bertins, I.Z., Panago, M., Badger, T.M., & Klibanski, A. (1980). Hypothalamic amenorrhea in runners of normal body composition. *Endocrine Research Communications*, **7**, 13-25.

Pohl, C.R., Richardson, D.W., Hutchison, J.S., Germak, J.A., & Krobil, E. (1983). Hypophysiotropic signal frequency and functioning of the pituitary ovarian system in the rhesus monkey. *Endocrinology*, **112**, 2076-2080.

Prior, J.C., Cameron, K., Yuen, B.H., & Thomas, J. (1982). Menstrual cycle changes with marathon training: Anovulation and short luteal phase. *Canadian Journal of Applied Sport Science*, **7**, 173-177.

Ross, G.T., & Hillier, S.G. (1978). Luteal maturation and luteal phase defect. *Clinical Obstetric Gynaecologica*, **5**, 391-409.

Schwartz, B., Cumming, D.C., Riordan, E., Selye, M., Yen, S.S.C., & Rebar, R.W. (1981). Exercise-associated amenorrhea: A distinct entity. *American Journal of Obstetrics and Gynecology*, **141**, 662-670.

Shangold, M., Freeman, R., Thyson, B., & Gatz, M. (1979). The relationship between long-distance running, plasma progesterone and luteal phase length. *Fertility and Sterility*, **31**, 130-133.

Shangold, M., & Levine, H.S. (1982). The effect of marathon training upon menstrual function. *American Journal of Obstetrics and Gynecology*, **143**, 862-869.

Sherman, M.B., & Korenman, S.G. (1974). Measurement of plasma LH, FSH, estradiol, and progesterone in disorders of the menstrual cycle: The short luteal phase. *Journal of Clinical Endocrinology and Metabolism*, **38**, 88-94.

Speroff, L., & Redwine, D.B. (1980). Exercise and menstrual function. *The Physician and Sportsmedicine*, **5**(8), 42-45.

Strott, C.A., Cargille, C.M., Ross, G.T., & Lipsett, M.B. (1970). The short luteal phase. *Journal of Clinical Endocrinology and Metabolism*, **30**, 246-251.

Wakat, D., Sweeney, K.A., & Rogol, A.D. (1982). Reproductive system function in women cross-country runners. *Medicine and Science in Sports and Exercise*, **14**, 263-269.

Warren, M.P. (1980). The effects of exercise on pubertal progression and reproductive function in girls. *Journal of Clinical Endocrinology and Metabolism*, **51**, 1150-1157.

Webb, J.L., Millan, D.L., & Stoltz, C.J. (1979). Gynecological survey of American female athletes competing at the Montreal Olympic Games. *Journal of Sportsmedicine and Physical Fitness*, **19**, 405-412.

Werlin, L.B., & Hodgen, G.D. (1983). Gonadotropin-releasing hormone agonist suppresses ovulation, menses, and endometriosis in monkeys: An individualized, intermittent regimen. *Journal of Clinical Endocrinology and Metabolism*, **56**, 844-848.

Wu, C.H., & Mikhail, G. (1979). Plasma hormone profile in anovulation. *Fertility and Sterility*, **31**, 258-266.

Yoshida, T., Hattori, Y., Suzuki, H., & Noda, K. (1979). Gonadotropin in follicular phase in women with luteal phase defect. *Tohoku Journal of Experimental Medicine*, **129**, 135-138.

Zaharieva, E. (1965). Survey of sports women at the Tokyo Olympics. *Journal of Sportsmedicine and Physical Fitness*, **5**, 215-219.

diZerega, G.S., & Hodgen, G.D. (1981). Luteal phase dysfunction infertility: A sequel to aberrant folliculogenesis. *Fertility and Sterility*, **35**, 489-499.

diZerega, G.S., Turner, C.K., Stouffer, R.L., Anderson, L.D., Channing, C.P., & Hodgen, G.D. (1981). Suppression of follicle-stimulating-hormone-dependent folliculogenesis during the primate ovarian cycle. *Journal of Clinical Endocrinology and Metabolism*, **52**, 451-456.

Reactions to Arend Bonen's Presentation

Reactor: Edwin Dale

We have to distinguish between clinical and physiological use of the term *normal*. Dr. Bonen's research shows that normalcy may not be the same entity both physiologically and clinically. In regard to the short luteal phase, let's not become shortsighted and focus only on progesterone. Estradiol levels are definitely diminished in the short luteal phase. Estradiol values are usually very high in the luteal phase but when they are suppressed, a short luteal phase occurs. Estrogens seem to change in their ratios. The Arizona study showed that estradiol declined when training, whereas estrone did not change. That change in ratio between estrone and estradiol indicates that the woman is being exposed to estrogen which is not physiologically as potent as the one which exists in the normal situation.

Discussion

Unknown: If we are going to study patients and compare amenorrheic to truly normally eumenorrheic women, we should all use the same part of the follicular phase. I suggest that we use the early follicular phase rather than the midfollicular phase.

Arend Bonen: I agree.

Jerilynn Prior: Rebar and coworkers noted an anticipatory rise in both testosterone and LH prior to starting acute exercise. Did you see that, and what are your thoughts on it?

Arend Bonen: Yes, we saw that in the study where we tried to monitor about 6 hours and 2 hours before exercise. Obviously, there is a neurogenic factor that seems to be responsible, but it's hard to quantify or deal with it.

Ralph Hall: It has been shown that liver blood flow is inversely proportional to oxygen consumption. The harder you exercise, the less clearance you will have of substances like testosterone. Thus, you would not expect testosterone levels to change very much unless you rehydrate after exercise.

Arend Bonen: That was my point in showing the clearance data with some of the studies. I suspect you are talking about long-term exercise. In intense shorter exercise, I don't think dehydration is a problem.

Alan Rogol: Do you have any thoughts about whether total testosterone tells you what's going on in case of endocrine excess syndromes? Also, has anyone looked at free testosterone levels?

Arend Bonen: The free hormone levels are obviously the physiologically significant ones. We are measuring totals (as do most people). Because of increasing body temperature during exercise and because of the way it is bound to the protein, presumably, you are then creating a free pool of the hormone even if secretion isn't changing. Just by the temperature-induced effect, the binding is loosened. Secondly, some of the work in The Netherlands has looked at free hormone concentrations. The concentrations change somewhat but you don't get more information than by simply measuring the totals.

Unknown: There have been some reports recently of short luteal phases in normally nonathletic women being associated with minimally higher prolactin levels. In these women, there was some modification of that pattern with Bromo-Criptine therapy. Do you think any of this may be related to a short luteal phase?

Arend Bonen: It may well be because the prolactin levels seen with trained women during exercise are getting fairly high, and people are speculating that those high levels, if they persist for quite some time, may be related to a short luteal phase.

Barbara Drinkwater: Dehydration does not occur in the first 10 to 15 minutes, but changes in plasma volume do. Greenleaf has shown quite well that at exercise levels of about 70% VO_2max, you can lose as much as 10 to 12% of the plasma volume in the first 10 to 15 minutes.

Arend Bonen: I should point out that we corrected for hemoconcentration in all our data.

Ann Loucks: Regarding previous comments about the neurogenic component, we should not forget that disruption with exercise may be taking place at the ovary. The ovary does have sympathetic innervation. Catecholamines may be involved. There is a difference in the response of amenorrheic runners compared to cyclic runners in the adrenal gland. Amenorrheic runners do not show an increase in cortisol, DHEA, or androstenedione as do cycling runners.

Chris Cann: Dr. Dale's comment about ratios has merit. We know that there is a significant amount of variability in hormone levels so that statistically, we are showing significant differences.

Unknown: Do prolactin measurements have to be obtained at basal conditions (rested and fasted) or may they be taken at any time?

Arend Bonen: The studies that we do certainly are under basal conditions.

Alan Rogol: One of the problems with doing any study with prolactin is that just sticking a needle in someone may double, triple, or quadruple their levels if they are really frightened. It is a very volatile hormone. With an indwelling catheter, the time to take a basal sample is usually 30 to 45 minutes after inserting the catheter. That may have been a problem with previous studies.

Arend Bonen: With any hormone, you probably ought to leave the catheter in about an hour to assume you are starting at basal condition. That's a very standard procedure.

Alan Rogol: I agree, but prolactin seems to be even more volatile than other hormones.

Edwin Dale: We really have come a long way in the field of amenorrhea as related to exercise. There has been an evolution from descriptive studies to more sophisticated studies. Future studies will become even more sophisticated with the use of indwelling catheters, infusions of medications, and the measurement of end-point parameters such as beta endorphins and other neurotransmitters. It's an exciting future.

7

The Therapy of Reproductive System Changes Associated With Exercise Training

Jerilynn C. Prior
Yvette Vigna
University of British Columbia

We have limited information about the physiology of menstrual cycle changes occurring with conditioning exercise on which to base judgment about therapy. The following recommendations and discussion are a clinical approach. The underlying assumption is that exercise-associated menstrual cycle changes are physiologic adaptations to the challenge that exercise places on the individual woman.

It is important to remember the patient is a partner in the decision-making process regarding her care. The only appropriate therapy implies the physician and woman have a good level of understanding and trust between them. The background of the clinical situation, the physician's understanding of the mechanisms involved, and an honest appraisal of what is known and not known are necessary before a final decision about therapy can be made. The woman makes the final decision. That decision is based on her knowledge of the changes in her own body, the best information she can gain from all sources, and the recommendations of her physician. Therapy should be practical, available, and affordable. Furthermore, it must aim to be physiologic and do no harm. Information about side effects and future risks must be sought by both the physician and the woman concerned.

This manuscript would not have been possible without the patient support and secretarial help of Hazel Netterfield. My appreciation to Drs. Basil Ho Yuen and Sheila Pride for intellectual stimulation and criticism.

The question of therapy calls up another issue. If the physician or patient believes that menstrual cycle alterations are not related to exercise or weight loss, then these changes must be viewed as a disease. This places the physician and the woman under a great deal of responsibility to exclude any serious problem. If a pituitary or hypothalamic problem is suspected to cause anovulation, expensive CT scanning of the head, multiple hormone assays, and other investigations are essential. However, if it is assumed that changes are the result of the body's adaptation to exercise, then a physiologic approach to therapy can be taken. Exercise intensity can be decreased, weight brought toward a more sedentary normal level for that individual, and the changes monitored. If this physiologic adaptation model is true, the cycle should become normal and ovulatory.

An aid to understanding potential menstrual cycle change in a physiologic context is to consider the age of the woman and her activity level (see Figure 1). For the first 10 years of reproductive life, anovulation may be normal. Therefore, the exercising postmenarcheal woman is more vulnerable to menstrual cycle alterations and more likely to become amenorrheic with intense activity. The mature athlete with normal ovulatory cycles will probably develop a short luteal phase or become anovulatory.

Figure 1

A diagrammatic description of the characteristic types of menstrual cycles and how they vary with the age and activity of the woman.

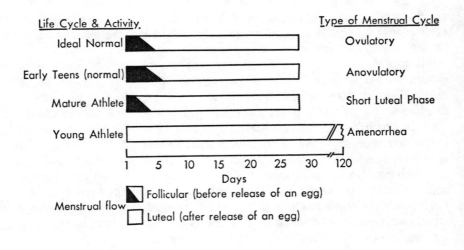

Definitions—The Normal Menstrual Cycle

A normal menstrual cycle must be clearly defined to judge the effectiveness of therapy. The following definitions are taken from several sources but mainly from the extensive work of Vollman (1977). He studied 691 women ranging in age at entry into the study from 4 to 63 years and gathered data on a total of 31,645 menstrual cycles. Using basal body temperature methods (BBT), he developed a quantitative, standardized way to interpret temperature data. His is the largest body of scientific data on the menstrual cycle and provides a useful tool to study exercise-related changes.

The normal intermenstrual interval, or cycle length, defined as the first day of bleeding up to, but not including, the onset of bleeding of the following cycle, is 21 to 36 days (Abraham, 1978; Vollman, 1977). A cycle of less than 21 days is polymenorrheic and one greater than 36 days is oligoamenorrheic. The follicular or postmenstrual proliferative phase of the cycle begins with the first day of bleeding and ends the day before ovulation occurs. It is defined by BBT methods as the first day of bleeding up to the temperature intercept (see Figure 2). Although the follicular phase is highly variable, the normal range is 10 to 20 days (Abraham, 1978; Vollmann, 1977).

The luteal or premenstrual secretory phase begins at ovulation and ends the day before onset of the next menstrual flow. However, pinpointing the exact time of ovulation is difficult. Multiple blood tests or ultrasound would be needed. Therefore, the luteal phase can be functionally defined as beginning with the thermal shift (or intercept) of the basal body temperatures. Vollmann (1977) lists the normal luteal phase as 10 to 16 days; Abraham (1978) defines it as 11 to 16 days. Vollman's definition is preferable because the methodology for determining the phase length is stated.

Symptoms associated with the ovulatory menstrual cycle include primary dysmenorrhea, molimina, and the premenstrual syndrome. Dysmenorrhea was originally ascribed to anger or fear concerning menstrual flow. It is now known that dysmenorrhea is caused by increased prostaglandin F_2 alpha production associated with increased uterine cramping and systemic effects (Dawood, 1983). Dysmenorrhea is usually limited to the ovulatory cycle and is improved after vaginal delivery, by oral contraceptives, or by antiprostaglandin agents (Dawood, 1983).

Premenstrual molimina are a collection of nondistressing symptoms serving as markers of the ovulatory cycle when they occur in a cycle of regular length (Maygar, Byers, Marshall, & Abraham, 1979). These symptoms include dysphoria with depression, anxiety or increased sense of stress, breast tenderness, changed appetite, and abdominal bloating or edema. These symptoms only occur in the luteal phase. A woman may also be aware she has

Figure 2

Diagram of the normal menstrual cycle divided by ovulation into two phases.

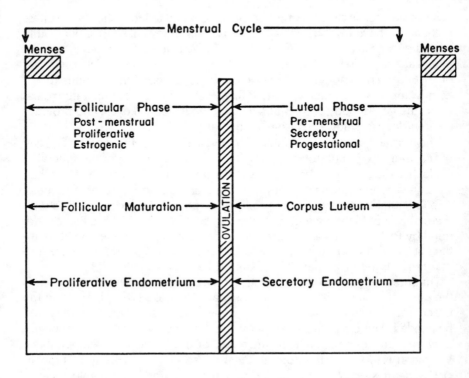

From "The normal menstrual cycle," by G.E. Abraham, 1978. In J.R. Givens (Ed.), *Endocrine causes of menstrual disorders*. Chicago: Year Book. Reprinted with permission.

ovulated by mild recognizable pain on one side of the lower abdomen (mittelschmertz) in the middle of the cycle. At midcycle there is a change from stringy clear mucus to watery cloudy mucus following ovulation (Maygar et al., 1979).

The premenstrual syndrome is a more intense experience of moliminal symptoms (Reid & Yen, 1983). These symptoms may be severe enough to interfere with daily life and work in more than 30% of normal women. Premenstrual symptoms, by definition, must occur in the luteal phase and be absent during the follicular phase. Dysphoric symptoms may be amplified by environmental and personal stress (see Figure 3). This syndrome probably has a complex hormonal etiology, though the psychoendocrinology is currently unknown (Reid & Yen, 1983).

Figure 3

Personal and environmental causes of stress which are not normally appreciated may cause symptoms when combined with the dysphoria of the premenstrual phase.

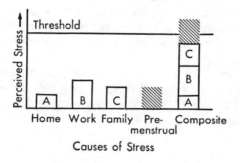

Causes of Stress

Definitions—Menstrual Cycle Alterations

Menstrual cycle changes associated with exercise need to be defined, so therapy can be appropriately given and effectively judged.

- *Inadequate corpus luteum* A short luteal phase of less than 8 days and infertility are usually part of the disorder known as inadequate corpus luteum (Jones, 1975). The diagnosis is normally made following an endometrial biopsy. The hormonal maturation of the lining of the uterus (endometrium) is sampled and documented to be either delayed, inappropriate for the age of the corpus luteum, or out of sequence within itself. Although the inadequate corpus luteum can be suspected from a short luteal phase or luteal progesterone levels, the diagnosis can only be definitively made by endometrial biopsy (Jones, 1975).
- *Anovulation* Anovulation is absence of egg release. In women with menstrual bleeding, anovulation is documented by a lack of thermal shift on basal temperature records and no progesterone rise premenstrually. There is no luteal phase. Population studies show that the usual cycle length of an anovulatory cycle is the same as that of a normal cycle, 21 to 36 days (Vollman, 1977). Anovulation is a hormonal state of unopposed estrogen and may increase risk of endometrial and breast cancer (Cowan, Gordis, Tonascia, & Jones, 1981; Speroff, Glass, & Kase, 1983).

- *Oligoamenorrhea*   Oligoamenorrhea means that menses occur at intervals of greater than 36 days (Abraham, 1977). Although most oligoamenorrheic cycles are anovulatory, a prolonged follicular phase may result in a longer cycle length with a normal ovulatory phase.
- *Secondary amenorrhea*   Secondary amenorrhea is defined differently by numerous authors and not defined by most. It has been defined as absence of menses for 6 months or no period for three of the usual cycle intervals (Speroff, Glass, & Kase, 1983). The best definition seems to be no menses in any consecutive 6-month period. Secondary amenorrhea is associated with low-estrogen levels.
- *Primary amenorrhea*   Primary amenorrhea means no menses by the age of 14 with no evidence of growth or secondary sexual development, or no period by the age of 16 regardless of growth and secondary sexual characteristics (Speroff, Glass, & Kase, 1983).

Therapy—Contraception

The first consideration in recommending therapy for the sedentary or athletic woman is to control fertility. The contraception used should not interfere with the chosen exercise, should not present complications, and should not suppress the normal hormonal control of the menstrual cycle. Ideal methods currently do not exist.

Barrier methods interfere least with the woman's hormonal system. The diaphragm, cervical cap, or condom must be used consistently and with adequate spermicidal jelly. An additional applicator of spermicidal jelly placed in the vagina is recommended after the mechanical barrier is in place. Evidence suggests that these measures, used conscientiously, are as effective as other reversible methods of contraception. Additionally, BBT monitoring could caution the woman about her time of increased fertility (days 10 to 18). If the luteal phase extends longer than 16 days, pregnancy must be suspected.

The oral contraceptive pill has been recommended as therapy. Although "the pill" controls fertility and provides adequate estrogen to prevent bone loss, potential thrombotic and cardiovascular risks (Stadel, 1981) and decreased exercise performance (Daggett, Davies, & Boobis, 1983) make it unacceptable to many health-conscious women.

Therapy—Conditions in the Normal Menstrual Cycle

Therapy for some conditions associated with a normal cycle may be appropriate. Dysmenorrhea can now be prevented in 80% of women by antiprostaglandin agents (Dawood, 1983). At the first sign of menstrual flow or cramping, these agents should be started and repeated at 3 to 4 hour intervals for the first 12 to 48 hours, until symptomatic relief is achieved. Naproxen sodium (275-mg tablets) is an effective member of the antiprostaglandin family of drugs.

Although premenstrual molimina does not require any therapy, the premenstrual syndrome may become quite severe (Reid & Yen, 1983). The following suggestions are based on clinical experience. Breast symptoms usually improve if caffeine is avoided and if vitamin B6 (Pyridoxine) is taken in pharmacologic amounts of 100 to 500 mg per day for the 2 luteal-phase weeks. If symptoms are severe, Bromocriptine, a dopamine agonist, can be given with food (1.25 to 2.5 mg at bedtime and breakfast). Side effects of Bromocriptine therapy include gastric irritation and nausea, which are lessened if the pill is taken with food, and postural hypotension.

Premenstrual symptoms related to fluid retention and bloating can be treated by avoiding high-salt foods and by decreasing the length of time during the day spent on the feet. Beginning a mild weight loss program will potentiate a physiologic diuresis. A diuretic is not indicated and should be avoided. Dysphoric symptoms during the premenstrual phase such as anxiety, depression, and irritability are often improved by knowledge that the symptoms are real and temporary. Acute exercise often improves this dysphoria.

The appetite cravings of the premenstrual phase can be satisfied by low-caloric foods such as carrots and celery or by frequent feedings of complex carbohydrates such as muffins, granola, crackers, whole-grain breads, or unsalted popcorn. If chocolate can be avoided, breast tenderness and fluid retention seem to be lessened. If overeating becomes unavoidable, it is preferable to indulge in bulky, healthy foods rather than concentrated simple carbohydrates. The woman should be warned that her alcohol tolerance may be lowered during this phase of her cycle.

Progesterone therapy has been advocated as a treatment for the premenstrual syndrome. Many authors advise doses which are pharmacologic and suppress ovulation. It can be given more physiologically as oral Provera (Medroxyprogesterone, 5 mg, two tablets per day on days 16 to 25). Although scientific evidence is lacking, many women experience subjective improvement. Preliminary work done in 1984 at our center shows that conditioning exercise decreases breast tenderness, fluid retention, and overall symptoms of the premenstrual phase.

Therapy—
Menstrual Cycle Changes Associated With Exercise

All menstrual cycle changes occurring with exercise are probably associated with a lower mean estradiol level. This was shown in prospective studies which did not characterize menstrual cycle change (e.g., Boyden, Pamenter, Stanforth, Rotkis, & Wilmore, 1983). Normal estrogen levels are important to build bone and prevent bone loss (Nordin, MacGregor, & Smith, 1966). Intense exercise may increase the risk of osteopenia (less bone) or early osteoporosis (fractures associated with less dense bone), especially if amenorrhea persists. This risk can be minimized by increasing calcium intake. The normal recommended dietary intake of calcium is 800 mg per day. If estrogen levels are low, the oral intake can be safely doubled and will probably prevent bone loss (Heaney et al., 1982). Each dairy product serving provides 200 mg of calcium (8 oz of milk, 4 oz of yogurt or cottage cheese, or 2 oz of hard cheese equal 200 mg calcium). It is practical to recommend oral calcium, 1 gm per day in addition to 4 dairy-product servings, or to take 1.6 gm of calcium supplement per day if dairy products are not preferred. Tums® is a readily available, inexpensive form of calcium carbonate providing 200 mg of calcium per tablet.

The inadequate corpus luteum should only be treated if fertility is desired. The first therapy is to decrease exercise intensity and achieve a normal weight. After the diagnosis is confirmed by endometrial biopsy, progesterone suppositories may be given vaginally, 25 mg in the morning and at bedtime for 12 days beginning on Day 14. This therapy will not interfere with fetal development. Progesterone is continued for 18 weeks after pregnancy is achieved.

Anovulation must be recognized and treated to prevent increased risk of endometrial and breast cancer (Cowan et al., 1981). The anovulatory cycle of normal length may be a common form of exercise-associated menstrual cycle change recognized by absence of molimina, no basal temperature plateau, and/or a low progesterone value (less than 5 mg/ml) the week before menses begin. Provera (5 mg, two tablets during days 16 to 25 for 10 days of each cycle) is the appropriate therapy (Stadel, 1981). Barrier methods for contraception are necessary because Provera can masculinize a female fetus. Oligoamenorrhea can also be treated with Provera for 10 days on a monthly basis. This will achieve regular, predictable cycles and prevent the risk of endometrial and breast cancer. The woman may prefer to take Provera for 10 days every 2 months so return of normal cyclic menses can be noted.

Secondary amenorrhea is the exercise-associated menstrual cycle disorder that has received the most publicity. First and foremost we must ensure that the woman is not pregnant. This can be done with a single estradiol level or pregnancy test. The first recommendation is to reverse any weight loss associated with exercise and to hold training at a steady moderate level (less than the maximum previously achieved). If menstrual flow does not return after 3 months, a further evaluation is necessary to rule out thyroid, pituitary, or psychologic abnormality. If serious problems are excluded and if exercise and lean body weight are an important part of the woman's lifestyle, then the role of therapy is to prevent the complications of low-estrogen levels. It is extremely important that calcium be supplemented, probably 1.6 to 2.4

gm of oral calcium a day. If vaginal symptoms interfere with sexual enjoyment or urethral symptoms occur (recurrent cystitis, obstruction, or frequency), local estrogen therapy with 1/2 applicator (2 gm) of conjugated estrogen vaginal cream (Premarin) taken one night a week often provides relief.

Delayed menarche or primary amenorrhea in the athletic teenager can be approached in the same way as secondary amenorrhea. Initially, a reversal of weight loss and a steady level of moderate training are necessary. If these measures do not result in increased sexual maturation, a growth spurt, or the onset of menses after 3 months, then further evaluation is needed.

If infertility is a problem, a basal temperature record will provide important information. It is important to achieve an ideal weight (which might be considerably heavier than the woman feels is appropriate for her athletic activity) and to decrease training to a moderate nonstressful level. If ovulatory menses do not occur after 3 months, further investigation of infertility should be initiated.

The appropriate therapy for menstrual cycle changes associated with exercise requires a clear understanding of the woman and her particular sport, and a good partnership and trust between the woman and her physician. Therapy is aimed at preventing any potential complications. The physiologic approach to these disorders suggests that decreasing exercise to a nonstressful level and increasing weight will cause a resumption of normal menses. Therapies can become more specific as further information on the etiology and hormonal mechanisms involved in menstrual cycle change with exercise is obtained.

References

Abraham, G.E. (1978). The normal menstrual cycle. In J.R. Givens (Ed.), *Endocrine causes of menstrual disorders*. Chicago: Year Book.

Boyden, T.W., Pamenter, R.W., Stanforth, P., Rotkis, T., & Wilmore, J. (1983). Sex steroids and endurance running in women. *Fertility and Sterility*, **3915**, 629-632.

Cowan, L.D., Gordis, L., Tonascia, J.A., & Jones, G.E.S. (1981). Breast cancer incidence in women with a history of progesterone deficiency. *American Journal of Epidemiology*, **114**, 209-216.

Daggett, A., Davies, B., & Boobis, L. (1983). Physiological and biochemical responses to exercise following oral contraceptive use. *Medicine and Science in Sport and Exercise*, **15**, 174.

Dawood, M.Y. (1983). Dysmenorrhea. *Clinical Obstetrics and Gynecology*, **26**, 719-727.

Heaney, R.O., Gallagher, J.C., Johnston, C.C., Neer, R., Parfait, A.M., Bchir, M.B., & Whedon, G.D. (1982). Calcium, nutrition and bone health in the elderly. *American Journal of Clinical Nutrition, 36,* 986-1013.

Jones, G.S. (1975). Luteal phase. In S.J. Behrman & R.W. Kirstner (Eds.), *Progress in infertility* (pp. 299-324). Boston: Little Brown.

Maygar, D.M., Byers, S.P., Marshall, J.R., & Abraham, G.E. (1979). Regular menstrual cycles and premenstrual molimina as indicators of ovulation. *Obstetrics and Gynecology, 53,* 411-414.

Nordin, B.E.C., MacGregor, J., & Smith, D.A. (1966). The incidence of osteoporosis in normal women: Relation to age and the menopause. *Quarterly Journal of Medicine, 35,* 25-38.

Reid, R.L., & Yen, S.S.C. (1983). The premenstrual syndrome. *Clinical Obstetrics and Gynecology, 26*(3), 710-718.

Speroff, L., Glass, R.H., & Kase, N.G. (1983). *Clinical gynecologic endocrinology and infertility* (3rd Ed.). Baltimore: Williams and Wilkins.

Stadel, B.V. (1981). Oral contraceptives and cardiovascular disease, parts 1 and 2. *New England Journal of Medicine, 305,* 612-618, 672-677.

Vollman, R.F. (1977). The menstrual cycle. In E.A. Friedman (Ed.), *Major problems in obstetrics & gynecology.* Toronto: W.B. Saunders.

Reactions to Jerilynn Prior's Presentation

Discussion

Jackie Berning: Being a nutritionist, my first inclination in talking about increasing calcium is to question the use of supplements. Optimal absorption of calcium occurs more rapidly and to a greater extent in whole foods than when a Tums is taken. Calcium carbonate absorption may be 40% with the Tums compared to 90 to 100% in foods. The recommended daily allowance for calcium is 800 mg; that's 2 glasses of milk a day, not counting calcium from other food groups. Increasing yogurt, ice cream, and all those other foods that are higher in calcium is a better approach than taking another pill because you also are getting lactose, vitamin D, and other compounds.

Jerilynn Prior: The general consensus is that we should provide calcium, including dietary calcium and whatever supplement may be needed, to reach 1.5 g a day.

Karen Nilson: Many of the runners and athletes we tell to take extra calcium are also on very high doses of other vitamins including vitamin D. Can we get ourselves in trouble by having high doses of vitamin D and calcium?

Jerilynn Prior: I agree, vitamin D more than 400 IU per day should be avoided.

Robert Marcus: What is the threshold for hypercalcemic conditions? I think there is clearly a risk when you get to doses of 10,000 units of vitamin D a day or more. Even bypassing the whole issue of increasing calcium and hypercalcemia, you do cause direct bone resorption. It's more risky for vitamin A. It is very common to find people taking as much as 50,000 to 100,000 units of vitamin A a day because they believe it will prevent them from getting cancer, from getting colds, and do all sorts of other things to their acne. vitamin A in high doses can directly cause bone loss as well. The point about hypervitamin doses is a legitimate concern.

8

Relationship Between Altered Reproductive Function and Osteoporosis

Barbara L. Drinkwater
Pacific Medical Center

Discussions of osteoporosis are usually set in the context of problems associated with aging or in relation to some pathological condition affecting bone metabolism. The possibility that healthy active young women may be subject to involutional bone loss as a byproduct of their exercise habits is disconcerting. Yet evidence is accumulating (Cann, Martin, & Genant, 1982; Drinkwater et al., 1984) that hypoestrogenic amenorrheic athletes are experiencing a decrease in vertebral bone mineral density (BMD). Although it is generally accepted that the low-estrogen levels found in postmenopausal women are associated with the high incidence of osteoporosis in that age group (Lindquist, Bengtsson, Hansson, & Roos, 1981), there was a tacit assumption that exercise, which appears to increase BMD in postmenopausal women (Smith, Reddan, & Smith, 1981), would protect the younger athlete. That postulate is now in question.

At present, many unanswered questions concern the etiology, prevention, and treatment of osteoporosis. The issue is complex because the mechanisms involved are complex. To understand how estrogen, exercise, and age might interact to affect bone mineralization requires a basic understanding of the bone remodeling process and how it varies with age.

Bone Remodeling

Bone is a metabolically active tissue whose structure is constantly remodeled through a sequence of bone resorption and bone formation. In the early adult years the two events are coupled so that each balances the other and bone mass remains constant. At some point during the fourth or fifth decade this process becomes uncoupled. Bone resorption exceeds bone formation leading to a gradual decrease in bone mass. In some individuals bone mass may eventually be reduced to a level at which structural failure occurs with little or no trauma. The majority of these individuals are postmenopausal women in whom morbidity and mortality related to osteoporotic fractures have now reached epidemic proportions.

A recent review by Raisz and Kream (1983) summarizes experimental data describing the regulation of bone formation at the molecular, cellular, and tissue level and discusses at what level and by what mechanism hormones and other factors might affect the remodeling process. They state that while much has been learned in recent years about how bone forms, the precise mechanisms by which the process is controlled are unknown. The effect of parathyroid hormone (PTH), for example, illustrates the intricate relationships involved. When serum calcium levels fall, PTH stimulates osteoclastic activity, thus mobilizing calcium from bone to reestablish normal serum calcium concentration. However, PTH has also been observed to stimulate bone formation. The apparent discrepancy in observations can be traced to different experimental protocols. The action of PTH on bone formation differs in vitro and in vivo, is dose dependent, and varies depending on whether infusion is intermittent or continuous (Heersche, 1982; Raisz & Kream, 1983; Tam, 1982).

Similar contradictions have been observed for other hormones, including estrogen. Because osteoporosis is the result of a negative imbalance between resorption and formation in the remodeling process, learning how hormones and other factors regulate bone formation is a critical first step in finding an agent that will restore balance or even reverse the imbalance to produce a net gain in bone mass. At present most treatments focus on decreasing the rate of bone turnover on the theory that if each remodeling cycle results in a net decrease in bone mass, slowing turnover rate will also slow bone loss (Parfitt, 1982).

All individuals lose bone mass with aging, but the effects of decreased skeletal density are more evident in women than in men. Colles fractures are 10 times more common in women over age 60 than in men (Hammond & Maxson, 1982). Hip fractures, a more serious problem, average 200,000 per year among older women, and approximately 30% of these are followed by complications leading to death (Avioli, 1981). Two models have been advanced (Lindquist et al., 1981) to explain the sex difference in incidence of osteoporosis. One assumes that both men and women lose bone at the same rate following skeletal maturity but that women reach the fracture threshold earlier than men because their initial bone mass is less. The second model holds that women lose bone at a faster rate than men, a rate which accelerates following menopause. Most experimental data support the latter model because of the close association of bone loss with estrogen deficiency. However, the two models are not mutually exclusive. Both the greater bone mass of males at peak skeletal maturity and a slower rate of loss may protect them against early osteoporotic fractures.

Even within gender there are differences between individuals. Not all postmenopausal women have pathological manifestations of osteoporosis (Stevenson & Whitehead, 1982). Slender caucasian women of northern European descent who lead sedentary lives and have an inadequate dietary intake of calcium appear to be most at risk (Hammond & Maxson, 1982; Lane & Vigorita, 1983; Parfitt, 1982; Stevenson & Whitehead, 1982). At present the interaction of these genetic factors and lifestyles with the bone remodeling process is not completely understood.

Concern for the amenorrheic athlete centers on the possibility that her hypoestrogenic status may initiate the uncoupling of bone formation and resorption and accelerate bone loss 10 to 20 years before it usually occurs. If so, the problem must be recognized and steps taken to find the most appropriate treatment for these young women.

Estrogen and Bone Mass

Most of what is known or hypothesized about the effect of diminished estrogen levels on bone comes from studies of women with reduced ovarian function as a result of aging, surgery, or disease (Cann, Genant, Ettinger, & Gordon, 1980; Dalen, Lamke, & Wallgren, 1974; Klibanski et al., 1980; Nachtigall, Nachtigall, Nachtigall, & Beckman, 1979; Schlechte, Sherman, & Martin, 1983). In each case, a decrease in estrogen is associated with a decrease in bone mass. There is a difference of opinion, however, about the type of bone—trabecular or cortical—most affected by estrogen withdrawal. Riggs et al. (1981) reported no marked bone loss from the appendicular skeleton (which is largely cortical bone) prior to age 50, but noted a steady decrease in the primarily trabecular bone of the spine from the early adult years onward. They conclude that estrogen deficiency has a more marked effect on cortical bone than on trabecular bone. In contrast, Parfitt (1982a) reports a rapid loss in trabecular bone in the first 3 to 5 years following menopause. The discrepancy may be related to the use of both linear and curvilinear regression analysis in the Riggs et al. data. A cubic function, the best fit for the data across ages 20 to 84, shows a peak BMD in the midradius at about age 36 and a continuous decline thereafter. Fitting the same data with two regression lines, one for ages 20 to 50 and another for ages 50 and over, indicated no change in BMD for the women in the 20 to 50 age bracket and a significant negative slope after age 50. However, fitting a linear regression line to curvilinear data can be expected to result in a slope not significantly different from zero, which may explain the apparent lack of any decrease in cortical bone during the 20 to 50 years age span. It appears more likely that the decrease in bone mineral content does not begin until the middle of the fourth decade.

When estrogen is abruptly withdrawn, as in the case of surgical menopause, there is little doubt that the effect is primarily on trabecular bone. Both Dalen et al. (1974) and Cann et al. (1980) recorded marked decrements in the mineral content of trabecular skeletal areas of oophorectomized women but not in cortical bone. In the Dalen et al. study a decrease in BMD was found in the distal radius, the third lumbar vertebra, and the neck of the femur 5 to 10 years following surgery. Cann et al. found a significant decrement in vertebral bone mass as early as 12 months following the operation and at the radial diaphysis by 24 months.

A decrease in bone density has also been reported (Klibanski et al., 1980; Schlechte et al., 1983) for young amenorrheic hyperprolactinemic women using a measurement site one third of the radius length proximal to the styloid process, an area which is primarily cortical bone. Klibanski et al. reported that the decrease in bone mass was directly related to the level of estrogen deficiency, but Schlechte et al. found no correlation between estradiol concentration and bone density. Because not all amenorrheic hyperprolactinemic women are hypoestrogenic, these authors suggest that excess prolactin, not estrogen deficiency, may account for the decrease in bone mass observed in these women. It is entirely possible that a decrease in estrogen or an increase in prolactin, with or without estrogen deficiency, might have differential effects on trabecular or cortical bone. Seeman et al. (1982) studied the effect of six endocrine disorders at three skeletal sites and concluded that the results of endocrine dysfunction on bone mass are disease and site specific. At present the weight of the evidence favors trabecular bone as the site where the effects of estrogen deficiency are most likely to be noticed.

Perhaps the most substantial evidence for a relationship between estrogen and bone mineral content comes from studies of the effectiveness of estrogen replacement therapy in halting bone loss in postmenopausal and oophorectomized women. A 2-year study by Recker, Saville, and Heaney (1977) examined the relative effectiveness of estrogen and calcium supplements and found that estrogen therapy was the more effective treatment in minimizing bone loss. An even more favorable response was noted by Jensen, Christiansen, and Transbøl (1982), who reported a significant *increase* in bone mineral content in 70-year-old women following 12 months treatment with an estrogen/gestagen agent. A similar protective effect has been reported by Lindsay, Hart, Forest, and Baird (1980) for oophorectomized women.

The mechanism by which estrogen exerts its protective effect is unknown. It is presumed that its role is indirect because no estrogen receptors have been found on bone (Hammond & Maxson, 1982). One possible mode of action involves an estrogenic effect on PTH activity, either by reducing the sensitivity of bone to PTH or directly suppressing PTH secretion (Aloia, 1982; Hammond & Maxson, 1982). The end result would be an inhibition of bone resorption and a decrease in bone loss. An alternate explanation involves the intestinal absorption of calcium. The administration of estrogen to postmenopausal women improves their calcium balance by increasing absorption and decreasing urinary excretion, possibly by increasing circulating levels of 1,25-dihydroxy-vitamin D (Hammond & Maxson, 1982).

There is some disagreement within the research community over the relationship between calcium intake and osteoporosis. Calcium balance, however, is clearly affected by estrogen deficiency. Heaney, Recker, and Saville (1978) have shown that postmenopausal women have a negative calcium balance that is approximately 24 mg/day greater than that of premenopausal women or a postmenopausal group treated with estrogen. They suggest that hypoestrogenic women may require a daily calcium intake of 1.5 g/day to remain in calcium balance while 1 g/day would be adequate for women with normal estrogen levels.

Exercise and Bone Mass

It has been well established (Aloia, 1982; Smith, 1981) that inactivity leads to calcium resorption from bone and that increased activity, such as that experienced by athletes, leads to greater bone density. The recent reports (Cann et al., 1982; Drinkwater et al., 1984) of a decrease in vertebral BMD among young amenorrheic athletes might suggest that exercise encourages bone hypertrophy in women only in the presence of estrogen were it not for reports (Smith, 1981) that involutional bone loss may be halted or even reversed in postmenopausal women not receiving estrogen therapy. Aloia, Cohn, Ostuni, Cane, and Ellis (1978) compared total body calcium and regional bone mass in 18 postmenopausal women, 9 of whom exercised three times a week for a year. The total body calcium of the active group increased 2.5% while that of the sedentary group decreased by 2.4%. In a larger sample of older women aged 69 to 95, Smith, Reddan, and Smith (1981) found that women who exercised increased bone mass by 2.29% over a 3-year period while the nonactive women lost an additional 3.29% of bone mineral content. For these elderly estrogen deficient women, physical activity was helpful in maintaining skeletal mass.

The mechanism by which exercise affects bone homeostasis may be central via improved circulation or local through mechanical stress applied directly to the bone (Smith et al., 1981). If the latter is the primary stimulus to bone hypertrophy, the effect of exercise on bone mineral content would be most apparent in those areas where muscular contraction and gravity provide the greatest stress. Both studies (Cann et al., 1982; Drinkwater et al., 1984) that reported a low-vertebral BMD in amenorrheic athletes have included primarily runners in their subject pool. While a decrease in vertebral bone mass may be a concern in itself, it does not negate a role for exercise in preserving or enhancing bone mineral content in areas under greater mechanical stress during running. The neck of the femur would be an excellent site to measure because it, like the vertebrae, is primarily trabecular bone. If additional data suggests that there is indeed a generalized decrease in bone mass in amenorrheic athletes, the implication will be that some factor which distinguishes the young hypoestrogenic female from the older estrogen-deficient woman affects the interaction between exercise and bone formation.

References

Aloia, J.F. (1982). Estrogen and exercise in prevention and treatment of osteoporosis. *Geriatrics, 37*, 81-85.

Aloia, J.F., Cohn, S.H., Ostuni, J.A., Cane, R., & Ellis, K. (1978). Prevention of involutional bone loss by exercise. *Annals of International Medicine, 39*, 356-358.

Avioli, L.V. (1981). Postmenopausal osteoporosis: Prevention vs cure. *Federation Proceedings, 40*, 2418-2422.

Cann, C.E., Genant, H.K., Ettinger, B., & Gordon, G.S. (1980). Spinal mineral loss in oophorectomized women. *Journal of the American Medical Association, 244*, 2056-2059.

Cann, C.E., Martin, M.C., & Genant, H.K. (1982). Detection of premenopausal amenorrheic women at risk for the development of osteoporosis. In Program and Abstracts of the 64th Annual Meeting of the Endocrine Society (p. 266). Baltimore: Wilkens and Wilkens.

Dalen, N., Lamke, B., & Wallgren, A. (1974). Bone mineral losses in oophorectomized women. *Journal of Bone and Joint Surgery, 56A*, 1235-1238.

Drinkwater, B.L., Nilson, K., Chesnut, C.H. III., Bremner, W.J., Shainholtz, S., & Southworth, M.B. (1984). Bone mineral content of amenorrheic and eumenorrheic athletes. *New England Journal of Medicine, 311*, 277-281.

Hammond, C.B., & Maxson, W.S. (1982). Current status of estrogen therapy for the menopause. *Fertility and Sterility, 37*, 5-25.

Heaney, R.P., Recker, R.R., & Saville, P.D. (1978). Menopausal changes in calcium balance performance. *Journal of Laboratory and Clinical Medicine,* **92,** 953-963.

Heersche, J.N.M. (1982). In vitro studies of bone formation and resorption. *Clinical Investigative Medicine,* **5,** 173-178.

Jensen, G.F., Christiansen, C., & Transbøl, I. (1982). Treatment of post menopausal osteoporosis. A controlled therapeutic trial comparing estrogen/ gestagen, 1,2-Dihydroxy-vitamin D_3 and calcium. *Clinical Endocrinology,* **16,** 515-524.

Klibanski, A., Neer, R.M., Beitins, I.Z., Ridgeway, E.C., Zervas, N.T., & McArthur, J.W. (1980). Decreased bone density in hyperprolactinemic women. *New England Journal of Medicine,* **303,** 1511-1514.

Lane, J.M., & Vigorita, V.J. (1983). Osteoporosis. *Journal of Bone and Joint Surgery,* **65A,** 274-278.

Lindquist, O., Bengtsson, C., Hansson, T., & Roos, B. (1981). Bone mineral content in relation to age and menopause in middle-aged women. *Scandinavian Journal of Clinical Laboratory Investigations,* **41,** 215-223.

Lindsay, R., Hart, D.M., Forest, C., & Baird, C. (1980). Prevention of spinal osteoporosis in oophorectomized women. *Lancet,* **2,** 1151-1157.

Nachtigall, L.E., Nachtigall, R.H., Nachtigall, R.D., & Beckman, E.M. (March 1979). Estrogen replacement therapy I: A 10-year prospective study in the relationship to osteoporosis. *Obstetrics and Gynecology,* **53,** 277-281.

Parfitt, A.M. (1982a). The contribution of bone histology to understanding the pathogenesis and improving the management of osteoporosis. *Clinical and Investigative Medicine,* **5,** 163-167.

Parfitt, A.M. (1982b). Treatment of osteoporosis: Theoretical possibilities. *Clinical and Investigative Medicine,* **5,** 181-183.

Raisz, L.G., & Kream, B.E. (1983). Regulation of bone formation, I. *New England Journal of Medicine,* **309,** 29-35.

Raisz, L.G., & Kream, B.E. (1983). Regulation of bone formation, II. *New England Journal of Medicine,* **309,** 83-89.

Recker, R.R., Saville, P.D., & Heaney, R.P. (1977). Effect of estrogens and calcium carbonate on bone loss in postmenopausal women. *Annals of Internal Medicine,* **87,** 649-655.

Riggs, B.L., Wahner, H.W., Dunn, W.L., Mazess, R.B., Offord, K.P., & Melton, L.J. (1981). Differential changes in bone mineral density of the appendicular and axial skeleton with aging. *Journal of Clinical Investigations,* **67,** 328-335.

Schlechte, J.A., Sherman, B., & Martin, R. (1983). Bone density in amenorrheic women with and without hyperprolactinemia. *Journal of Clinical Endocrinology and Metabolism, 56,* 1120-1123.

Seaman, E., Wahner, H.W., Offord, K.P., Kumar, R., Johnson, W.J., & Riggs, B.L. (1982). Differential effects of endocrine dysfunction on the axial and the appendicular skeleton. *Journal of Clinical Investigations, 69,* 1302-1309.

Smith, E.L. (1981). Bone changes in the exercising older adult. In E.L. Smith & R.C. Serfass (Eds.), *Exercise and aging* (pp. 179-186). Hillside, NJ: Enslow.

Smith, E.L., Reddan, W., & Smith, P.E. (1981). Physical activity and calcium modalities for bone mineral increase in aged women. *Medicine and Science in Sports and Exercise, 13,* 60-64.

Stevenson, J.C., & Whitehead, M.I. (1982). Postmenopausal osteoporosis. *British Journal of Medicine, 285,* 585-588.

Tam, C.S. (1982). Hormonal control of bone formation in vivo. *Clinical and Investigative Medicine, 5,* 169-172.

Reactions to Barbara Drinkwater's Presentation

Discussion

Harmon Brown: Is there any information which suggests that in this age group, the enhancement of calcium intake (absorption) may be able to overcome some of the bone mineral changes that you see because you are dealing with a complex of low estrogen (perhaps) and deficient calcium intake? I think we should ensure that the women are not going to take estrogen replacements and that they should take at least 1,200 to 1,500 mg of calcium per day.

Barbara Drinkwater: Almost all women are calcium deficient. So I don't see how one can go wrong in following the suggestion to increase calcium intake. But in terms of estrogen replacement therapy, please note that at least in our study, not all of our amenorrheic women were low in bone density.

Edwin Dale: So as a blanket statement you cannot say that an amenorrheic athlete is necessarily going to be deficient in bone. You actually have to go in there and take a look and find out if they are. There are a couple of things in looking at the studies relating estrogen to bone mineral density that were of some concern. One is what happens when you stop estrogen therapy? Is it necessary that they have the therapy every month? Would stimulation at more infrequent intervals be sufficient? What is the sufficient dose for stimulation for the amenorrheic athlete? There's an awful lot we need to know about the interaction of estrogen replacement therapy (ERT) with bone mineral density in this age group before we want to suggest estrogen replacement as a blanket prescription. One thing that concerns me is the possibility that young, amenorrheic athletes (or the coach or parents) reading about this situation may start prescribing Premarin without the aid of a physician. A mother may be sharing her pills with her daughter. We want to be very careful that we don't give the impression that this is something you can take on lightly.

Leonard Calabrese: You both (Drinkwater and Marcus) have some divergent data but your comparisons have been between amenorrheic and normally menstruating female runners only. What brought both of you to make the leap of faith to look at only these groups? Why wasn't there a sedentary, age-matched, height-matched control group? Stress fractures of the lower extremities in athletes are not restricted to females. In one male dancer, we have seen a bizarre seven or eight stress fractures in one lower extremity. What about the other variables and what about your thoughts on other controls?

Barbara Drinkwater: I think you have a good point, and I will give you two reasons why we did what we did. One was money—we didn't have the funds. The second reason was time on the dual photon.

Jackie Puhl: Dr. Marcus, you gave the impression that because your subjects were taking iron supplements and were meeting two thirds of their RDA that their iron intake was satisfactory and supplements were not needed. I don't believe that's true. First, the RDA is probably a little low to adequately meet iron needs, particularly for the women runners, because there appears to be an iron cost associated with running training. Unless you have substantiated iron status with blood test results, you don't know if iron supplements are needed or not.

Chris Cann: From cross-sectional data, women who have been amenorrheic for perhaps 1 to 3 years have significantly more bone than those who have been amenorrheic for 5 to 10 years. We know there is a relatively rapid phase of bone loss. But we also know that the ones that have been amenorrheic for 5 years are not lower or higher in bone density than ones that have been amenorrheic for 10 or 20 years. It appears that most of the bone is lost in the first few years.

Robert Marcus: A gram of vitamin C will almost double estrogen levels in the blood, so you have to be careful the subjects are not on vitamin C when you evaluate estrogen.

Wayne Sinning: Concerning efficiency, there are considerable data on efficiency of runners, at least in males. The average runner uses about .73 C per pound of body weight per mile run. The trained person uses just slightly over .7 C. Based on that information, I calculated that there must be quite a difference between amenorrheic and normally cycling individuals. Amenorrheics are expending about 500 C a day for running whereas cycling women would be using 290 to 300 C per day. So there is quite a difference in energy expenditure and daily energy requirements on the basis of the 25 miles and the 43 miles you gave us.

Michelle Warren: The issue that you raised today about the calorie deficiency brought on by the physical activity is very important. I have a pet theory about amenorrhea. I feel it is due to a relative energy drain, not just training effects. We should take very careful exercise histories and calculate the amount of calories that have been expended, just the way we have taken a careful nutritional history. It would add a lot to our understanding of the problem.

Ed Burke: We have done detailed diet analyses of our women cyclists during competition. We found the same interesting conclusions (low calorie intake) during actual competition. We knew they were very accurate records because a dietician worked and ate with the team. But you have to be careful with elite athletes because when they are not training or competing they are very lethargic, do very little, and put out very little energy.

9

New Medical Imaging Technology: Can We Really Use It in Sports Medicine?

Christopher E. Cann
University of California at San Francisco

Measurements are of prime importance in sports. On the field, distance and time are quantified with extreme accuracy. Off the field, body mass, size, composition, and performance characteristics are continually monitored. For such quantitative measurements, advances in technology have always made a significant impact. In the last several years, medical technology has made several major advances both in imaging techniques and tissue composition analysis, but much of this new methodology has not been accessible to the community outside of clinical medicine. Only recently has the newer instrumentation been available on a relatively widespread basis for investigational purposes as clinical demands have become less intense. As the new modalities have become available, new methods for both monitoring and diagnosis have started to be adapted from the clinical sphere to the special needs of sports medicine.

Body Composition Analysis

One area of investigation which has been easily adapted from clinical studies is that of body composition analysis. This includes such diverse elements as bone and muscle mass, muscle, lung, and fat volumes, and the distribution of bone and muscle as a function of exercise regimen. In addition, the newer techniques have been refined to the point that their sensitivity to change in these diverse parameters is 5 to 10 times better than older methods, so new areas of investigation have become accessible. Where previous studies required change with a factor of two or more in relatively large populations to show longitudinal changes in exercise programs, new methodology can be adapted to provide sensitivity to a few percent change in an individual subject for various measurements. However, in instituting new measurement techniques, we must be able to cross-calibrate our results with the older methods so that we can properly interpret the changes we see in the perspective of the larger body of previous research.

Several new techniques using currently available clinical instruments can be adapted directly to the study of body composition and noninvasive measures of tissue physiology. These include quantitative computed tomography (Q CT), nuclear magnetic resonance imaging (MRI), nuclear magnetic resonance spectroscopy (NMR), and single photon and dual photon absorptiometry (SPA, DPA). In addition, neutron activation analysis (NAA) has been used as a research tool in this area. The adaptation of these methodologies is straightforward, in principle, but interpretation of results can often be difficult. In clinical medicine, one generally wishes to diagnose or monitor an abnormal condition, where in preventative or sports medicine we monitor the normal age-related or adaptive changes of the body to a variety of stimuli. It is in this context that the use of the new technologies will be considered.

The new technology discussed here can be divided generally into methods which provide three-dimensional or cross-sectional information, often with the additional feature of a cross-sectional or omniplanar image (Q CT, MRI, NMR), or linear and two-dimensional projection methods which generally are not used for imaging but are optimized for specific measurements (SPA, DPA, NAA). To understand the utility, advantages, and disadvantages of each methodology, a basic knowledge of how each works and what each can deliver is useful.

Single Photon Absorptiometry

Single photon absorptiometry was first developed by Cameron and Sorensen (1963) as a method to measure the quantity of bone mineral in a long bone. It is best known through the clinical application of the Norland-Cameron Bone Mineral Analyzer, a commercial instrument first marketed in the late 1960s. More recently, a device manufactured by Mölsgard and based on a modification of single-scan SPA has been introduced into the U.S. and Europe, providing a significant improvement in bone measurement reproducibility. Photon absorptiometry is based on the fact that bone mineral absorbs more x-rays or gamma-rays than does soft tissue (the reason bones are white on standard x-rays) and that the amount of bone in the path of the radiation beam is quantitatively related to the attenuation or absorption of the radiation. Both commercial devices use small radiation sources of 125_I which emits low-energy gamma rays. These photons are collimated to a small beam a few millimeters wide which is passed across the bone to be measured (radius, ulna, or tibia, surrounded by a water bag or water bath). A detector on the opposite side of the bone counts the photons which come through. By comparing the number of photons coming through the bone with those coming through only soft tissue and through a calibration standard, the quantity of bone through which the beam passed is calculated. The instrument is calibrated so that the amount of bone is expressed as grams of mineral per 1 cm length of bone.

The method is simple and straightforward to quantify the amount of bone *at the measurement site*. The measurement of mineral content in the long bones can be used to predict total body mineral content in normal subjects relatively well. However, it is not very useful in monitoring the effects of treatment or other stimulus on the skeleton because the cortical (compact) bone measured changes so slowly in response to a stimulus that it usually takes 2 to 3 years to see a change. SPA is relatively widely available at modest cost.

Dual Photon Absorptiometry

Like SPA, dual photon absorptiometry has been developed primarily for bone mineral measurement (Krolner et al., 1980; Riggs et al., 1981). It uses the same principle as SPA, measuring total bone mineral in the path of the beam but scans in a rectilinear fashion over a large region, usually the spine, femoral neck, or the whole body. The use of two gamma-rays instead of one eliminates the need for the water bath (constant tissue thickness); thus a subject can be scanned in air while lying on a table. The main advantages of this technique over SPA for body composition analysis are the ability to measure total body mineral directly (with the proper instrument) and to measure regional bone mass in areas such as the spine where a relatively high proportion of metabolically active trabecular bone (50 to 60%) increases the sensitivity to change in response to a stimulus. Disadvantages include limited availability and increased cost relative to SPA.

Neutron Activation Analysis

Direct measurement of the elemental composition of the body by in vivo neutron activation analysis has been used to estimate the mass of bone, muscle, and fat (Cohn & Dombrowski, 1971). However, the limited availability of this method (one center), the cost, and the high radiation dose limit its usefulness for most studies.

Quantitative Computed Tomography

In contrast to the above methods which were developed for specific purposes (primarily in bone), Q CT, MRI, and NMR are outgrowths of the development of new general diagnostic modalities in radiology based primarily on imaging. Computed tomography as an imaging modality in many ways revolutionized diagnostic radiology. The cross-sectional display of anatomy afforded by this technique provides the means whereby an isolated region can be examined free from surrounding tissue which overlies the region of interest (ROI) in a conventional radiograph. However, the pictorial display of the CT image has overshadowed the basis of that image, which is in reality a map of x-ray attenuation values for points in a cross-sectional region of the body. CT is basically an extension of SPA; instead of obtaining a profile of attentuation measurements along a line a few millimeters wide, however, a series of profiles is obtained from different "view" angles. By a mathematical process known as backprojection, these profiles are then used to generate a two-dimensional map of tissue x-ray attentuation (see Figure 1).

These attenuation values when properly interpreted contain information about the chemical composition of the tissues and, along with the image, can be used to measure organ volumes and body compartments such as bone, muscle, lung volume, and fat directly (see Figure 2) (Cann, Martin, Genant, & Jaffe, 1984; Grauer, Moss, Cann, & Goldberg, 1984; Heymsfield et al., 1979; Termote, Baert, Crolla, Palmers, & Bulcke, 1980). Because each CT scan is normally only 5 to 10 mm thick, it would be difficult to do total body scans for many individuals. However, it is possible to scan at selected sites and use an algorithm to predict body composition. Q CT has also been used to measure the densities of tissue, the size of discrete muscle groups, and other parameters related to musculoskeletal function and is generally done with a radiation exposure 10 to 50 times less than that used for diagnostic CT imaging purposes. To date, Q CT has been somewhat restricted because of limited access to CT scanners and the cost of obtaining time. This is changing because over 3,000 machines are now available in the U.S., many in private clinics, and new applications are being developed for CT to more fully utilize the instrumentation.

Magnetic Resonance Imaging

Magnetic resonance imaging is a departure from conventional imaging modalities in radiology in that it does not use ionizing radiation but depends instead on relatively high strength magnetic fields (.1 to .5 Tesla) and radio waves to produce a signal. Radiography depends on the physical characteristics of a tissue such as the number of electrons and the average atomic number

---

Figure 1

Schematic representation of the basis of computed tomography (CT). CT involves two primary steps: (a) projection, or collection of data, and (b) backprojection, or the processing of the data mathematically to reconstruct an image of the original object. Left: Objects in a box are "viewed" by x-rays from two different angles, and the transmission of x-rays through the objects is recorded on a film or x-ray detector. The area under the curve of transmitted intensity is proportional to the size and density of the objects. SPA and DPA use the equivalent of the projection step to measure bone mineral content in the radius and spine. Right: Backprojection attributes the measured intensities equally to a series of points along each line in the original box. When this is done from the two different angles, spatial localization of the original objects is achieved. Present day commercial CT scanners view objects and backproject from 300 to 1000 angles, providing a reconstructed image in which typically 0.5 to 1.0 mm objects are resolved.

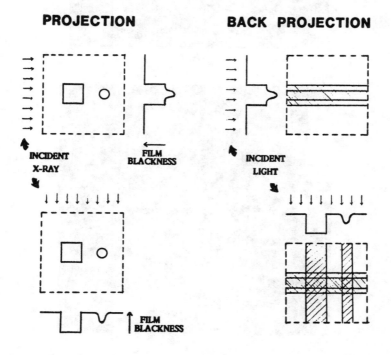

Figure 2

Quantitative CT measurement of various body compartments. Scans are normally done at 1/10 to 1/50 the normal x-ray exposure used for CT imaging. A) Vertebral trabecular mineral content is measured by comparing the CT number in the center of the vertebral body to a bone reference calibration standard. Total mass and volume of bone in a vertebra is measured in a similar

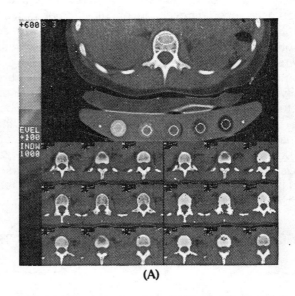

(A)

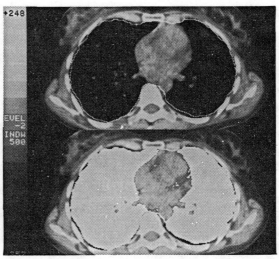

(B)

Figure 2 (Cont.)

manner by summing all pixels which contain bone. B) Lung volume and density at expiration is obtained by scanning rapidly at 2 to 3 cm intervals (1 scan/5 seconds). C) Size and density of isolated muscle groups in the leg are measured directly. D) Body fat is measured directly based on its lower density (therefore lower CT number).

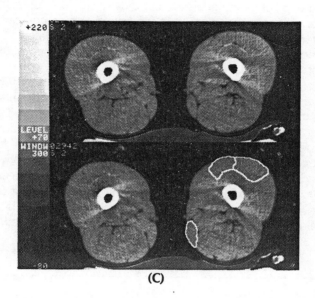

(C)

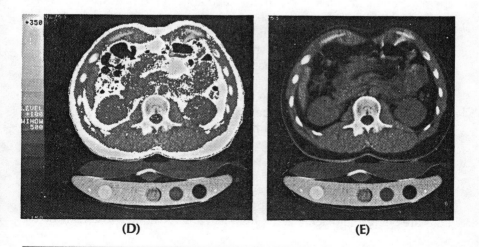

(D)   (E)

of the atoms in the tissue (calcium and phosphorus in bone have high atomic number; carbon, oxygen, and hydrogen in soft tissue have low atomic number) to produce the variations in signal that we see.

MRI depends in part upon the physical characteristics of the tissue (the number of protons) but also in part on the chemical interactions between the protons in that tissue. Because the protons (hydrogen nuclei) act like little magnets, their interactions will depend on how close they are to each other and also on what other materials are close by to shield these magnets from one another. For example, protons in fat, bound to a central carbon atom, will act differently than protons in water bound to oxygen atoms. Thus, with proper choice of scanning parameters we can optimize the visualization of one type of tissue over another.

As in CT, MRI provides a cross-sectional display of anatomy such that we can distinguish size of muscle groups and layers of fat; however, because MRI scans take minutes to complete, this technique is limited in its ability to measure such things as lung volume because of respiratory motion. In addition, because bone is a solid and contains few protons (therefore, low signal), we cannot use MRI to measure the amount of bone in the body. To date, MRI has had its greatest success in neurologic imaging and, because of its sensitivity to water, in disorders where edema is signifcant. At the present time, access to MRI is limited to several research centers but this should improve within the next year as more MRI scanners are marketed.

Nuclear Magnetic Resonance

Perhaps the greatest potential of the new technology in sports medicine is the emergence of nuclear magnetic resonance spectroscopy to study the chemical composition and functional capabilities of various tissues. Where MRI is limited to proton images because of its lower magnetic field strength, NMR at 1 to 2 Tesla field strength has the capabilities for both imaging and spectroscopy of hydrogen, carbon, phosphorus, and other less abundant elements such as sodium. NMR has for years been the organic chemists' tool for studying molecular structure, and each chemical compound has its own characteristic NMR spectrum. Initial work with in vivo NMR included work in laboratory animals and in human limbs because the only magnets available with high enough field strengths had a small hole for samples.

Recently, instrumentation has become available which combines the high fields necesary for spectroscopy (1.5 to 2 Tesla) with large apertures and imaging capabilities. This now opens the door for local tissue physiology studies, using the image to localize the region to be studied and the spectroscopic capabilities to study tissue function. At the present time, whole-body NMR units are being manufactured and installed, and it will be 1 to 2 years before the instrument capabilities are brought to their full potential. Because of expense, these units will not be as available as CT or MRI units; however, for properly designed research protocols it is expected that limited time will be available.

Future Research

These newer technologies may have a significant impact in several areas of sports medicine and physiology. Clinically, stress fractures are generally diagnosed from a bone scan rather than from plain x-rays, and it is difficult to determine the size of a fracture or the extent of healing. High quality CT scans at the site of injury may be useful in showing minor soft tissue inflammation before the blood flow changes show up on a bone scan; MRI may also be useful in this regard because of its sensitivity to edema. Screening of amenorrheic athletes for bone loss is best done by Q CT (Cann et al., 1984), which is also the most sensitive method for monitoring therapy. Diagnosis of cruciate tears or meniscal tears in the knee may be done by CT without invasive techniques such as arthrography or arthroscopy (see Figure 3).

Specific physiologic and morphologic changes associated with exercise can be studied with the newer techniques. Currently under investigation using Q CT is the effect of muscle development with exercise on the density of bone at ligamentous and tendon insertions in the leg and posterior spinal elements in runners and weightlifters. In addition, direct measurement of body fat distributions and lung volumes in individuals can be compared with skinfold thickness and hydrostatic weighing in vivo to better define the parameters measured with these techniques and refine the algorithms used to determine lean body mass. It may be possible with MRI to determine the state of the endometrium in amenorrheic or anovulatory athletes and to correlate serial MRI scans with hormonal and body temperature profiles. With the advent of NMR, direct in vivo measurement of tissue pH and lactate buildup in muscle with exercise may be done, as well as direct determination of phosphorus metabolism. It may even be feasible to measure glucose utilization and storage using fluorine-labeled glucose or deoxyglucose compounds like those used in nuclear medicine.

Exercise physiology is very different from clinical medicine. On the one hand we deal with patients in whom there is a disruption of the normal homeostatic state of the body, and the diagnosis and treatment of this disorder is of paramount importance. On the other hand we are concerned with a healthy individual in whom the homeostatic systems are presumably intact, and we are studying the normal adaptive responses of the body to stresses

Figure 3

A) 1.5 mm thick CT scans through the knee joint of a patient with a suspected right meniscal or cruciate tear. A bucket handle tear is seen in the right medial meniscus, compared to the normal contiguous crescent of cartilage seen on the left side. The diagnosis in this case was proven at arthroscopy. B) A series of 1.5 mm thick contiguously spaced scans were done and reformatted in the sagittal plane to demonstrate the cruciate ligaments (intact).

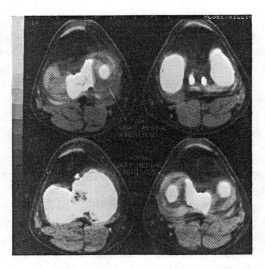

(A)

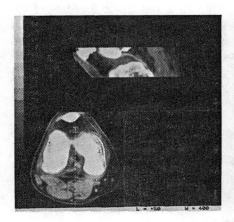
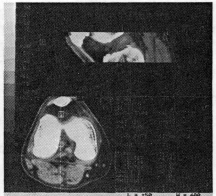

(B)

on this system. In a properly functioning homeostatic system, the responses we see may be slight, so we must not only know where to look for the most sensitive response, but how to ask the proper question, make the proper measurement, and interpret the data we obtain. If we do not design our experiments properly, all the new technology in the world will not help us to understand the fundamental responses of the system that we study.

References

Cameron, J., & Sorensen, J. (1963). Measurement of bone mineral in vivo: An improved method. *Science*, **142**, 230-232.

Cann, C.E., Martin, M.C., Genant, H.K., & Jaffe, R.B. (1984). Decreased spinal mineral content in amenorrheic women. *Journal of the American Medical Association*, **251**, 626-629.

Cohn, S.H., & Dombrowski, C.S. (1971). Measurement of total body calcium, sodium, chlorine, nitrogen and phosphorus in man by in vivo neutron activation analysis. *Journal of Nuclear Medicine*, **12**, 499.

Grauer, W.O., Moss, A.A., Cann, C.E., & Goldberg, H.I. (1984). Quantification of body fat distribution in the abdomen using computed tomography. *American Journal of Clinical Nutrition*, **39**, 631-637.

Heymsfield, S.B., Fulenwider, T., Nordlinger, B., Barlow, R., Sones, P., & Kutner, M. (1979). Accurate measurement of liver, kidney and spleen volume and mass by computerized axial tomography. *Annals of Internal Medicine*, **90**, 185-187.

Krolner, B., Pors Nielsen, S., Lund, B., Lund, B.J., Sorenson, O.H., & Uhrenholdt, A. (1980). Measurement of bone mineral content (BMC) of the lumbar spine: II. Correlation between forearm BMC and lumbar spine BMC. *Scandinavian Journal of Clinical Laboratory Investigations*, **40**, 665-670.

Riggs, B.L., Wahner, H.W., Dunn, W.L., Mazess, R.B., Offord, K.P., & Melton, L.J. (1981). Differential changes in bone mineral density of the appendicular and axial skeleton with aging. Relationship to spinal osteoporosis. *Journal of Clinical Investigations*, **67**, 328-335.

Termote, J.-L., Baert, A., Crolla, D., Palmers, Y., & Bulcke, J.A. (1980). Computed tomography of the normal and pathologic muscular system. *Radiology*, **137**, 439-444.

Reactions to Christopher Cann's Presentation

Discussion

Joel Stager: During this symposium it has been suggested that there seems to be a plastic period and that if you intervene within a critical period, you may have a good chance of recovery of some of this bone loss. Is there a good theory for that or is that sort of a guess?

Chris Cann: The basis for that is all the data we have on either post-menopausal or perimenopausal women in an estrogen deficient state. Bone turnover in response to any metabolic stimulus is a transient phase which increases and then drops back to normal. Estrogen has a protective effect on bone. You remove it, bone resorption increases dramatically.

Edwin Dale: We have to be very rigorous about controls in any new technology. Also, to have a control group that is age 40 and an amenorrheic group that is age 23 or 30 is not appropriate. Comparing groups widely distant in terms of weight is also not appropriate. We know weight is a factor in bone density. Let's not start publishing data that's going to confuse people. We also have a responsibility to be very honest about radiation dose. It's one thing to send somebody who's got a very possible stress fracture for a technicium scan; they've got a disease. It's another thing to test somebody who does not have a disease. I hope that in your published paper you will tell us the quantal dose, the machine you're using, when it was updated, and when it was tested.

Chris Cann: In terms of dose, we measured less than 3 millirem gonadal exposure and less than 100 millirem to 3 inches of the abdomen for the CT scan. From the standpoint of using a particular technique, we do have to be very precise. Also, I think we're starting to come up with enough data now that the possibility of a predisposition to a pathologic condition 20 or 30 years from now is also a clinical problem.

10

Problems in Methodology

Anne B. Loucks
University of California at San Diego

This paper concerns important methodological issues in research on the relationship between the menstrual cycle and physical activity. Of the many issues, only those will be stressed that are most important in determining the reliability of experimental results. The objectives of this paper are first to encourage discussion of these issues in the hope that by consensus the differences in methodology that may have contributed to conflicting results in the past can be resolved, and second, to increase the probability that future results will be reliable, consistent, and informative.

Although the relationship between the menstrual cycle and physical activity may initially seem to be a narrow topic, it actually encompasses a wide range of subtopics that include (a) normal disruptions of the reproductive system such as menarche, pregnancy, and menopause, (b) abnormal disruptions such as primary and secondary amenorrhea, oligomenorrhea, and luteal phase deficiency, (c) possible consequences such as infertility and osteoporosis, (d) effects of pharmaceuticals such as contraceptives, anabolic steroids, and anti-inflammatory drugs, (e) the age-old issue of dysmenorrhea and other effects of the menstrual cycle upon athletic performance, and (f) the manipulation of the menstrual cycle for the purpose of improving performance. Each of these topics alone could be the basis for a career in research: Our knowledge is inadequate in every one of them.

Athletes, coaches, physicians, and parents impatiently ask scientists about the incidence of abnormalities in athletes, about their reversibility, about possible consequences, about diagnostic procedures, about physiological mechanisms, and about the effectiveness and side effects of various treatments. The amount of work required to answer all these questions is staggering, and the work has just begun. Scientists have volunteered to try to answer these questions: Because it is our responsibility to answer them correctly, it is our job to design and conduct our experiments rigorously.

Limitations on Research

Scientific enquiry into the menstrual cycle and physical activity may be limited by a number of conditions that can obstruct an experiment entirely or influence its outcome even more than measurement techniques or strategies of experimental design. Several of these conditions are discussed below.

The State of Knowledge
About the Female Reproductive System

An inescapable limitation on research on the menstrual cycle and physical activity is the state of knowledge about the female reproductive system. Many people are under the illusion that the regulation of the female reproductive system is well understood and that researchers merely need to make a few measurements in order to correctly identify the particular physiological mechanism of athletic amenorrhea. The opposite is much closer to the truth: Only through intensive research on athletic amenorrhea can the female reproductive system be understood. How can investigators of menstrual disruption in athletes, for example, assess the impact of hormonal changes during exercise when reproductive endocrinologists have not yet determined the durations of hormone concentrations required for end organ responses? Are we to interpret differences in hormone concentrations between amenorrheic and cyclic athletes as causes or as effects of reproductive disruption? Bluntly, the effects of physical activity upon the regulation of the menstrual cycle are *not* known, and because the answers to many questions about the menstrual cycle and physical activity are beyond the frontier of knowledge about the regulation of the female reproductive system, investigators of these questions must be prepared to do fundamental research on female reproduction.

An Interdisciplinary Problem

A second condition determining the success of reproductive research on athletes is the interdisciplinary nature of the problem. Real problems rarely fit tidily into abstract academic disciplines, and the effect of physical activity upon the menstrual cycle is no exception. Among nonathletes, strong evidence indicates that the menstrual cycle is affected by diet, psychological stress, and certain drugs. Physical activity itself and body composition have also been proposed to affect the female reproductive system. Reproductive experiments may call for hormone concentrations and bone mineral to be measured, drugs to be administered, or tissue samples to be obtained. Therefore, this research spans at least physiology, human performance, psychology, nutrition, endocrinology, radiology, and medicine. By contrast, individual scientists are typically experts in part of one academic discipline with a working familiarity with statistics. One must doubt at the very beginning, therefore, whether an individual scientist is capable of conducting reliable research in this area: Very likely, proper experimental controls and the collection and evaluation of all data relevant to a specific question dictate a multidisciplinary team approach.

In practice, unfortunately, multidisciplinary research teams almost immediately encounter interpersonal problems regarding communication, respect, and cooperation. Conflicts arise over language, priorities, ownership of data, sharing of costs, scheduling of tests, and other issues. These problems are emotionally unpleasant; the tendency is to avoid them by restricting the scope of the experiment and doing it alone. Because the reproductive system is so susceptible to so many factors, however, I do not see how the multidisciplinary team approach can be avoided without seriously compromising the merit of the study.

Subject Availability and Cooperation

A third condition underlying reproductive research on athletes is the availability and cooperation of experimental subjects. The best experimental design is useless without subjects. In general, the more demanding an experiment, the more difficult it is to recruit subjects and to be confident of their compliance with an experimental protocol, especially during unsupervised periods. Athletes are not like medical patients who may have desperate motivations to risk new treatments. Instead, they have little willingness to do anything that may interfere with their training or reduce their performance. This is especially true of trained control subjects who have no reason to be anxious about their condition. Investigators complain of athletes being uncooperative, irresponsible, and temperamental. In turn, athletes complain of investigators interfering with their workout schedules, subjecting them to distressing experimental procedures, treating them like guinea pigs, and neglecting to inform them of experimental results: Basically, they feel their needs and desires are not respected. If an experiment is to be successful, investigators need to anticipate these problems and accept that they may need their subjects much more than their subjects need them.

The goodwill of subjects must be nurtured, not just for the present experiment, but in anticipation of future ones also. Nevertheless, empirical compromises introduced to encourage subjects to volunteer may undermine the credibility of results, whether they are correct or not. On critical methodological issues, investigators must be willing to keep searching for subjects as long and as far as necessary.

Human Subjects Committee Approval

A precondition for almost all of this research is Human Subjects Committee approval. In some cases experiments involving drug administration, tissue sampling, or other risks to the health of the subject may be disapproved. Because Human Subjects Committees protect the privacy as well as the health of subjects, reproductive system researchers may be prohibited from enquiring about prior pregnancies, abortions, venereal diseases, or other aspects of menstrual and medical history relevant to the selection of subjects and the evaluation of data. Note that the issue here is not whether subjects are willing to answer the questions, but whether the investigators are permitted to ask them.

Political Concerns

Finally, the political context in which this research is conducted cannot be ignored. Women have struggled for decades for access to athletic facilities, and this struggle is not yet complete. In addition, only recently has the inclusion of physical activity in the concept of femininity become widespread among women. Some proponents of women's athletics fear that publicity about possible harmful effects of athletic training upon the female reproductive system may hinder this struggle or discourage this social change. In some cases, these fears are well founded. On the basis of insufficient evidence, New York State, for example, has prohibited competition in interscholastic athletic events by girls who have not attained menarche (Brody, 1982). Investigators must resist such overreaction by refusing to allow their tentative and inadequately substantiated hypotheses to be prematurely put forth as facts for the determination of public policy. Matters of medical treatment, public policy, and personal lifestyle should be based on knowledge, not on ideology— whether archaic ideology or new ideology—nor on incomplete research. Nevertheless, anxiety about the unwarranted application of experimental results cannot be allowed to obstruct the study of women's physiology: Investigators must never fail to perform an experiment out of fear of what they might discover.

Experimental Design

Experimental design is the basis for the logical structure of a scientific experiment. The validity of conclusions drawn from experimental observations depends upon correct experimental design. Several aspects of experimental design deserve emphasis when considering research on the menstrual cycle and physical activity: the susceptibility of a question to empirical observation; the explicit definition of terms; subject selection criteria; the capabilities and limitations of data collection techniques; and the interpretation of statistical results. These issues determine whether scientific experimentation is possible at all; whether it will use animals or humans as subjects; how subjects will be selected and allocated to experimental groups; whether the experiment will be prospective or retrospective, descriptive or mechanistic; and what conclusions can and cannot be drawn from the results.

The Susceptibility of the Question to Empirical Observation

Some questions about the menstrual cycle and physical activity may not be susceptible to empirical observation: The means of collecting the relevant data may not exist, or the necessary experiment may be logistically unfeasible. One example may be the question of the possible influence of premenarcheal training upon the age of menarche. Without sets of identical twins raised in the same households, one member of each set trained and the other not trained, can anyone be confident that, without training, two groups would have attained menarche at the same age? The logistics of a lengthy study of a sufficiently large number of sets of twins make this study highly unlikely to be organized or successfully conducted. Some questions, however important they may be to some people, simply cannot have scientific answers. In any case, the first step in experimental design is to be sure that the question of interest is susceptible to empirical observation.

Explicit Definition of Terms

Explicit quantitative definitions are essential to good experimental design and to clear publication of results. The absence of such definitions leads to large standard deviations in a given experiment and to results which conflict with those of other studies. Inconsistent definitions from study to study undermine the ability to compare their results and confuse both investigators and the public. Many terms basic to the study of the menstrual cycle and physical activity have been inadequately or inconsistently defined in the past: terms as basic as *amenorrhea, trained,* and *runner.* Of course, a single definition for all studies is not necessary or even desirable; for example, there is no correct definition for "amenorrhea." Nevertheless, *some* definition must be stated explicitly, along with the reason for using that definition in the particular experiment. If results are to be compared to previous findings, the same definition must be used as was used previously.

In the past, amenorrhea has been either completely undefined or variously defined as absence of menses for 3, 4, 6, 10, and 12 months, and as no more than one menses in the prior 10 months, or three menses in the past year. Much of the variability in incidence of amenorrhea from study to study is due to this variability in definition. Because studies of the incidence of secondary amenorrhea in the general population have used the 3-month definition for amenorrhea (Bachman & Kemmann, 1982; Pettersson, Fries, & Nillius, 1973; Singh, 1981), only those studies of the incidence of secondary amenorrhea among athletes which used the 3-month definition can validly compare the relative incidence of secondary amenorrhea among athletes and the general population. On the other hand, in a cross-sectional study of the effect of athletic amenorrhea on bone mineral content, the limited resolution of bone density measurement techniques may require a definition of amenorrhea as absence of menses for 1 or even 2 years in order for cumulative differences to be detectable. We should agree upon the definitions to be used for various experimental purposes: for determining incidence, for detecting osteoporosis, and for establishing that a transition from cyclic to acyclic status has occurred, to cite a few examples.

Subject Selection Criteria

Another major cause of variability within and between experiments is subject selection. This issue is ignored rather than resolved by permitting subjects to select themselves. Self-selection is notorious for skewing experimental results. Criteria for inclusion in a study and for assignment to experimental groups must be explicitly stated and related to the purpose of the study. Then this descriptive data must be reported so that the reader knows what was done to whom.

In studies of the effect of physical activity upon the menstrual cycle, only subjects whose menstrual cycles were altered after they began athletic training are appropriate. Several control groups may be needed for results to be correctly interpreted. In studies of athletic amenorrhea, for example, both trained and untrained cyclic control groups are needed to distinguish training effects that alter reproductive control from those that do not. This requires, of course, that the ovulatory status of all subjects be confirmed.

A procedure for selecting and allocating subjects may be more elaborate than the experiment itself, but the scientist cannot avoid it any more than the physician can avoid screening new patients. In both cases, the assignment of a patient or subject to a treatment or experimental group is based on extensive questionnaires, which must be clarified through personal interviews, and a workup that may involve pulmonary and cardiovascular function tests, blood tests, body composition measurements, and psychological and nutritional tests.

Capabilities and Limitations of Questionnaires

Questionnaires can serve three useful purposes in research on the menstrual cycle and physical activity. They can provide descriptive information on large groups of women; indeed, some information such as menstrual history can only be collected by means of questionnaires. Wherever feasible, however, information should be collected via a prospective daily record rather than by retrospective recollection. Questionnaires can also help to screen experimental subjects, although here physiological measurements and personal interviews are needed to confirm uncertainties. And, questionnaires can suggest physiological experiments. Questionnaires alone, however, cannot demonstrate a physiological mechanism because questionnaires cannot make physiological measurements.

The Interpretation of Statistical Results

One of the first problems that arises in designing an experiment is determining the number of subjects required to test for statistical significance. Another frequent difficulty in physiological research is the interpretation of the physiological importance of statistically significant differences. In studies of the female reproductive system, this difficulty is compounded by our ignorance about the physiological importance of differences in hormone concentrations. In the absence of this knowledge, the best approach to all three of these problems is to express differences between groups in terms of the normal range in the general population. Then the number of subjects needed to test for statistical significance can be calculated from the chosen significance criterion, the desired power of the test, and the number of population standard deviations that will be regarded as a physiologically important difference between groups; then, also, statistical significance and physiological importance will be equivalent (Beyer, 1968).

When interpreting statistical results, almost all investigators recognize intellectually that correlation does not imply a causal relationship; nevertheless, they are all inclined to treat correlations as if they actually are causal. Nor does a significant difference between means of descriptive characteristics imply a causal relationship in a physiological mechanism; but again investigators are inclined to interpret these differences as causally related to the basis for separating groups. Some studies, for example, have interpreted differences in fatness between amenorrheic and cyclic athletes as evidence that body fatness is involved in the mechanism of athletic amenorrhea. Some have recognized that the distribution in fatness in both groups overlap so much that only an individual critical fatness for maintenance of menses is tenable; but on the basis of overlapping descriptive data alone, individual variability in a critical fatness threshold looks exactly the same as the absence of any causal relationship at all between fatness and menstrual function. The only way to establish a causal relationship between fatness and menstrual function is via a controlled mechanistic study in which fatness is varied and effects upon the reproductive system are demonstrated endocrinologically. The study of the menstrual cycle and physical activity yearns for such mechanistic experiments.

Measurement Techniques

On the basis of experience and familiarity with the scholarly literature, an investigator of the menstrual cycle and physical activity will identify the parameters relevant to a particular scientific question for screening subjects and for the experiment itself. A study of thermoregulation in amenorrheic athletes, for example, must be controlled for those physiological conditions, such as body composition and aerobic capacity, which have been shown to affect thermoregulation: Only then can a further influence of reproductive status on thermoregulation be discerned.

The following four questions arise:

1. Are techniques available for measuring the relevant parameters directly in humans in vivo?
2. If no direct measurement is available for use with humans in vivo, are the empirical sacrifices in indirect measurements so great that the study must be performed by direct means in animal models or in vitro?
3. If acceptable methods are available for use in humans in vivo, what are the advantages and disadvantages of the various techniques for each particular parameter?
4. How are these techniques performed in order to minimize measurement error?

To ensure that measurements are within an error tolerance consistent with the inferences that are to be made, the conscientious investigator will answer these questions thoroughly before selecting any particular measurement technique.

The types of parameters relevant to research on the menstrual cycle and physical activity might be categorized as pertaining to endocrine status, the ovarian cycle, body composition, training, nutrition, psychological condition, histology, and medical and menstrual histories. Questionnaires can provide information on some of the parameters in some of these categories, but even in these categories additional important information can only be gathered by personal interviews or laboratory tests. Because the proper procedures for all of the techniques relevant to this research cannot be described here, the balance of this paper is concerned wih general measurement issues that the investigator of the menstrual cycle and physical activity must resolve for confidence in the data to be warranted.

Endocrine and Neuroendocrine Parameters

In most cases, endocrinologists are not able to make direct measurements in humans in vivo of the endocrine and neuroendocrine parameters controlling the reproductive system. These parameters include hormone concentrations and conversions at the target tissues, receptor concentrations on target membranes, and secretion rates. Instead, endocrinologists measure hormone and binding globulin concentrations in peripheral blood. The relationships between these concentrations in peripheral blood and cellular mechanisms in target tissues is not established. To some extent, these mechanisms can be investigated in humans in vivo by pharmacological means: Administration of catecholamine and opiate agonists and antagonists are examples. For the most part, however, this work will be done with human cells in culture or on animal models. Without the results of this basic research using direct methods, indirect studies of particular problems performed on humans in vivo cannot firmly identify altered mechanisms of reproductive control. Without knowledge of how these mechanisms are altered, precise diagnostic, preventative, and therapeutic procedures cannot be defined.

At present, indirect measurements of endocrine and neuroendocrine parameters are the best available basis for clinical evaluation of reproductive disorders and for the scientific evaluation of speculations about the control of the reproductive system. The accurate representation of endocrine status by measurement of hormone concentrations in peripheral blood requires the reduction of variability due to menstrual, diurnal, and pulsatile rhythms, plasma volume shifts, and environmental factors. Without these controls, endocrine data cannot be regarded as reliable.

The Ovarian Cycle

Assessment of the ovarian cycle entails two types of issues: adequacy and timing. Adequate gonadotropin stimulation and follicular development are necessary for ovulation and for the corpus luteum and endometrium to support a pregnancy. Menstruation is only the most superficial symptom of reproductive function: Its presence does not necessarily imply ovulation, and its absence does not necessarily imply anovulation. Therefore, more data is required to determine ovulatory status. Basal body temperature alone is not a reliable indicator of ovulation, because many women display no thermogenic response to progesterone (Bauman, 1981). Ovulation is usually inferred from measurements of progesterone, but, in fact, no lower threshold is well defined as a reliable sign of ovulation. Ovulation may be more reliably inferred if daily measurements near midcycle reveal an LH peak. Ultimately, the occurrence of ovulation may be demonstrated directly by ultrasonography.

Proof of luteal sufficiency is a pregnancy successfully carried to term. The next strongest evidence is provided by endometrial biopsy. Progesterone measurement alone cannot demonstrate endometrial responsiveness to hormonal stimulation, and individual variation in progesterone concentration is so great that no single level can be relied upon as either necessary or sufficient (Shangold, Berkeley, & Gray, 1983).

These conditions have several implications for research on the menstrual cycle and physical activity. First, a control group of menstruating athletes cannot be assumed to be ovulatory. Second, basal body temperature is not a reliable indicator of ovulation. If blood sampling for the LH peak and ultrasonography are unfeasible, then confidence in ovulation depends upon a conservatively high midluteal phase progesterone criterion. In studies of athletic amenorrhea, subjects who do not satisfy this criterion must be rejected; in studies of luteal phase deficiency, more information is required to classify these subjects properly.

Body Composition

Because direct measurement of body composition by dissection is impossible with human subjects in vivo, all body composition measurements utilize indirect techniques. The most accurate single indirect method is densitometry (measuring underwater weight and lung volumes), in which the experimental error is $\pm 3\%$ of body weight (Siri, 1956). Compared to densitometric measurements, methods based on height and weight (Keys & Brozek, 1953), anthropometry (Johnston, 1982), skinfold (Flint, Drinkwater, Wells, & Horvath, 1977), and predicted total body water (Loucks, Horvath, & Freedson, 1984), yield errors which are undesirable in scientific research and intolerable when applied to clinical problems. By combining densitometry and hydrometry, in which total body water is measured, experimental error can be reduced to less than $\pm 2\%$ of body weight (Siri, 1956). Most of the remaining error is due to uncertainty in the relative proportions of protein and mineral in nonfat body solids. Because statistically significant differences less than experimental errors cannot be regarded as meaningful, and because differences in fatness between experimental groups are often small in studies of the menstrual cycle and physical activity, the combined densitohydrometric method provides the soundest basis for inferences about any possible relationship between body composition and the menstrual cycle.

Psychological Condition

Psychological stress is known to disrupt the female reproductive system (Wentz, 1977). It has been surmised that athletic women experience more psychological stress than nonathletic women and that this stress is responsible for the greater incidence of reproductive dysfunction in athletes than in nonathletes. For these reasons, the psychological condition of subjects in studies of the menstrual cycle and physical activity should be determined as part of the screening process.

Despite this suspicion, however, repeated applications of standardized psychological tests have found amenorrheic and cyclic athletes to fall within the normal range of every psychological parameter tested (Schwartz et al., 1981; Galle, Freeman, Galle, Huggins, & Sondheimer, 1983; Gray & Dale, 1983). This leaves three possibilities:

1. Psychological stress may play no important role in reproductive dysfunction in athletes.
2. The standardized psychological tests utilized to date may not be sensitive enough to detect the small differences in psychological condition which may affect the reproductive system in athletes.
3. The tests may have been administered at the wrong time, that is, during a persistent reproductive dysfunction but after recovery from psychological stress.

Which of these possibilities is correct? Psychologists and psychiatrists need to be recruited into this research for this issue to be resolved.

Nutrition

Only the most superficial and inconclusive attempts have been made to investigate dietary associations with reproductive dysfunctions among athletes and the general role of diet in the control of the reproductive system. Again, the absence of basic knowledge will make inferences from the results of nutritional studies on female athletes all the more difficult to substantiate. Therefore, methodological precautions are especially important if nutritional data is to be at all useful. Data should be collected by dietary record rather than dietary recall, over as many days as is feasible, and during a period representative of the normal lifestyle. Efforts should be made to help subjects estimate dietary intake as accurately as possible. Because we do not know what nutritional factors—such as total caloric or protein content, specific amino or fatty acid, vitamin, or mineral deficiencies, or food additives—may be involved, data should be analyzed as extensively as can be afforded. Finally, evidence exists to suggest that sustained caloric deficiency leads to a reduction in metabolic rate (Stein, Schluter, & Diamond, 1983). Therefore, thyroid activity and metabolic rate should be measured as part of an evaluation of caloric sufficiency as well as to assess possible direct effects of metabolic rate upon the reproductive system via such measurements as hormone clearance rates and thyroid participation in regulation.

Physical Training

Because their level of physical activity is more easily quantified, participants in sports such as running, swimming, and cycling are more easily screened and matched than participants in sports such as gymnastics and dance. For control purposes, therefore, studies of gymnasts and dancers should select experimental and control subjects from the same team or company. Maximal aerobic power provides a physiological criterion for screening and matching purposes but, because of its large genetic component, should not be the sole indicator of the extent of physical training.

There are no well-defined categories of such a continuous parameter as the extent of physical training. Yet, to reduce variability in investigations of the effect of physical activity upon the menstrual cycle, investigators should try to select subjects from one portion of the full range of physical activity in which women are engaged. I suggest the following admittedly vaguely defined categories as representative of different degrees of physical activity and types of athletic lifestyle:

1. elite athletes—those competing on a national or international level;
2. competitive athletes—those competing locally, and who continually strive to improve their performances;
3. committed athletes—noncompetitive athletes whose intense training is a permanent part of their lifestyle; and
4. recreational athletes—those whose participation is fashionable and occasional, or regular but not strenuous.

To increase the likelihood that an effect of physical activity upon the reproductive system will be observed, if it exists, only elite and competitive athletes should be studied. The other groups may be useful, however, in other types of studies of the reproductive system, or for establishing incidences at those levels.

As with diet, a training record is a more reliable data base than a recollection of past training. When studying the hormonal response to exercise, three types of exercise are possible: uncontrolled, self-paced exercise; controlled, submaximal exercise; and a maximal aerobic power test. Investigators should choose the type of exercise appropriate to the question they are addressing. In addition, interpretations should not be based upon single blood samples drawn during intervals when hormone concentrations are changing rapidly.

Conclusions

Our ability to answer many questions about the menstrual cycle and physical activity is limited by our lack of knowledge about the regulation of the female reproductive system. The relationship between physical activity and the menstrual cycle is a multidisciplinary problem requiring a team approach for its investigation. Investigators need to be careful to consider the extent to which questions are susceptible to empirical observation, to define terms precisely and appropriately, and to screen and describe subjects thoroughly.

For this research, questionnaires alone are not sufficient, and the limitations of laboratory techniques also need to be recognized. To prevent many temporal and environmental influences from confounding endocrinological data, the collection of this data must be carefully controlled. Menstruation cannot be relied upon as the sole proof of unaltered reproductive function, and body composition cannot be determined accurately without densitometry. We may not know how to assess the effect of psychological factors upon the menstrual cycle. In contrast, many unutilized techniques are available for investigating the effect of dietary factors upon the reproductive system. In all of these studies, the level of physical activity needs to be quantified and controlled. Finally, to reiterate, the available indirect endocrinological methods are capable of providing data that can contradict or serve as a basis for hypotheses about the physiological mechanisms linking the menstrual cycle and physical activity; however, proof of these mechanisms will come only through basic research and new technologies for the more general study of the female reproductive system.

References

Bachman, G.A., & Kemmann, E. (1982). Prevalence of oligomenorrhea and amenorrhea in a college population. *American Journal of Obstetrics and Gynecology*, **144**, 98-102.

Bauman, J.E. (1981). Basal body temperature: Unreliable method of ovulation detection. *Fertility and Sterility, 36,* 729-733.

Beyer, W.H. (1968). Number of observations for t-test of difference between two means. In W.H. Beyer (Ed.), *Handbook of tables for probability and statistics* (2nd ed.) (pp. 286-287). Cleveland, OH: Chemical Rubber Company.

Brody, J.E. (1982, September 1). Effects of exercise on menstruation. *The New York Times,* pp. C1, C6.

Flint, M.M., Drinkwater, B.L., Wells, C.L., & Horvath, S.M. (1977). Validity of estimating body fat of females: Effect of age and fitness. *Human Biology, 49,* 559-572.

Galle, P.C., Freeman, E.W., Galle, M.G., Huggins, G.R., & Sondheimer, S.T. (1983). Physiologic and psychologic profiles in a survey of women runners. *Fertility and Sterility, 39,* 633-639.

Gray, D.P., & Dale, E. (1983). Variables associated with secondary amenorrhea in women runners. *Journal of Sport Sciences, 1,* 55-67.

Johnston, F.E. (1982). Relationships between body composition and anthropometry. *Human Biology, 54,* 221-245.

Keys, A., & Brozek, J. (1953). Body fat in adult man. *Physiological Reviews, 33,* 245-325.

Loucks, A.B., Horvath, S.M., & Freedson, P.S. (1984). Menstrual status and validation of body fat prediction in athletes. *Human Biology, 56,* 383-392.

Pettersson, F., Fries, H., & Nillius, S.J. (1973). Epidemiology of secondary amenorrhea. I. Incidence and prevalence rates. *American Journal of Obstetrics and Gynecology, 117,* 80-86.

Schwartz, B., Cumming, D.C., Riordan, E., Selye, M., Yen, S.S.C., & Rebar, R.W. (1981). Exercise-associated amenorrhea: A distinct entity? *American Journal of Obstetrics and Gynecology, 141,* 662-670.

Shangold, M., Berkeley, A., & Gray, J. (1983). Both midluteal serum progesterone levels and late luteal endometrial histology should be assessed in all infertile women. *Fertility and Sterility, 40,* 627-630.

Singh, K.B. (1981). Menstrual disorders in college students. *American Journal of Obstetrics and Gynecology, 140,* 299-302.

Siri, W.E. (1956). The gross composition of the body. In J.H. Lawrence & C.A. Tobias (Eds.), *Advances in biological and medical physics* (Vol. IV) (pp. 239-280). New York: Academic Press.

Stein, T.P., Schluter, M.D., & Diamond, C.E. (1983). Nutrition, protein turnover, and physical activity in young women. *American Journal of Clinical Nutrition*, **38**, 223-228.

Wentz, A.C. (1977). Psychogenic amenorrhea and anorexia nervosa. In J.R. Givens (Ed.), *Endocrine causes of menstrual disorders* (pp. 87-113). Chicago, IL: Year Book Medical Publishers.

Reactions to Anne Loucks' Presentation

Discussion

Anne Loucks: What are your ideas and thoughts on criteria for amenor-rhea that are appropriate for osteoporosis detection?

Barbara Drinkwater: In deciding on our criteria, we were concerned first of all with the sensitivity of the measuring instrument and the theoretical decrease that we might expect to see or the difference between amenorrheic and eumenorrheic groups. For that, we depended upon the results that Chris Cann found when he calculated out that the approximate decrease per year was 12%. The dual photon is quite capable of picking that up. We felt that a criterion of being amenorrheic for one year, with the possibility that this would cause the difference of 4.5% between groups, would be sensitive enough for us to find a difference, if in fact it existed. Our group average was 3.5%. The other thing to consider is the variability in the group. We all need to not only look at the alpha level of our test but the beta as well. One of the big reasons for so much variability on results and physiological data is that some people start out with such a small N. When considering the vari-ability, they don't have a prayer of finding a difference. Then the papers come out and say there was no difference. From the literature or pilot studies you should have a feel for the variability of the data that you are looking at and then you can come up with a physiologically meaningful difference. Then you can calculate the sample size that you need to have a reasonable chance of detecting that difference, if in fact it exists. In our study, we found a power better than 0.9 with an N of 14. If you do the same test with an N of 4, you don't have a chance of finding a significant difference.

Chris Cann: I'm biased toward longitudinal tests because the variability in a population is always going to kill you if you're looking at small numbers.

Finding a control group is sometimes very difficult. If you are able to work with technology that gives you data over a 1- or 2-year period, your longitudinal data will give a much more sensitive measure.

Anne Loucks: What definition is appropriate for determining that a transition from acyclic to cyclic status has occurred in a longitudinal study?

Jerilynn Prior: I think the most practical way to do it is with the basal body temperature which has been validated in numerous studies.

Unknown: If you're going to put a person in an acyclic group, there has to be some length of time (some criteria) that they've been acyclic. I think Dr. Prior made a good statement that you have to have some kind of systematic evaluation. You also have to have some kind of endocrinological evaluation. Somewhere along the line you have to measure a hormone to make sure you know that not only is the woman cyclic or acyclic, but is she ovulatory? Many women who haven't had any menstrual cycles for months become pregnant—and that means there was ovulation. I think we must have a standard definition—some sort of minimal, essential criteria. Then people may become more stringent depending on the question they want to ask. We need to use subjective, objective, and endocrine definitions.

Anne Loucks: What laboratory measurements are necessary to complement dietary analysis in studies of the menstrual cycle and physical activity?

Robert Marcus: The first thing is to get a registered dietician who knows the field in terms of ferreting out information and doing a nutritional assessment. Second, get some money to invest in a nutritional dietary analysis program for a microcomputer. It is also important to have some measure of metabolic rate. Serum triiodothyronine is probably the most accurate hormonal measurement for this. With just routine clinical chemistry, serum albumin is a reasonable, inexpensive measure; however, I think it falls apart unless you're dealing with profoundly malnourished hospitalized patients with a variety of illnesses.

One useful measurement is creatinine, using a 2-hour collection of urine, and then extrapolating to a 24-hour creatinine excretion value. In general, athletes have a high excretion of creatinine which is reflective of their lean body mass. Another measure is 3-methyl-histidine. Looking at various micronutrients can be a problem. None of the water-soluble vitamins is amenable to a simple lab test which will really tell you what the patient/subject's status is. They are often tedious and costly and not worth doing. The only water-soluble vitamin where a simple serum measurement does correlate pretty well with nutritional status is ascorbic acid. Vitamin A can also be measured in a simple serum assay and is not that difficult or expensive to do. Red blood cell folate has replaced plasma folate. It is not that expensive and is a very good index of folic acid status. Because folate is so abundant in a variety of vegetables, cereals, grains, and so forth, it is often a good sign of the general nutritional status. I would not waste the money to do a serum B-12 because the chances of picking up somebody with pernicious anemia are small.

Beverly Bullen: Hopefully, on a 3-day diet record we're getting at least 2 week days and 1 weekend day. I think it is necessary to see if there have been changes in their dietary habits over time, particularly relating to training. We felt that in order to follow people through training, it was necessary to really weigh their foods and have them calculated every day. Depending on the nutrients you want to follow, you might look at the particular laboratory test that would be necessary.

Michelle Warren: I am really concerned about the energy expenditure involved. I think it's important to look at the $\dot{V}O_2$max, BMR, the body temperature and thermogenic response to exercise, and diet (because athletes may differ in terms of their response). Body fat is still very important. I think we should keep open to simpler methods than the traditional body density methods.

Index